THE COMPETE
TRAEGER
WOOD PELLET GRILL AND SMOKER

THE EASY RECIPES FOR THE MOST FLAVORFUL

AND DELICIOUS BARBECUE

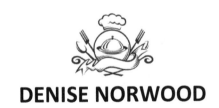

DENISE NORWOOD

CONTENTS

INTRODUCTION

What Exactly Are Wood Pellets?

Wood pellets are made from a combination of hardwood shavings and sawdust. This is pressurized, compressed down, and held together through the use of the wood's lignin, an all-natural binding agent. It's made into long, pencil-thick rods that are broken into smaller pieces. Most wood pellet pieces will be about a half-inch long.

During the compression of the wood shaving and sawdust mixture, most of the air and moisture is removed. Also, this mixture means you won't be burning any bark, dirt, etc that you would find on raw wood logs. This results in an extremely efficient and clean-burning fuel source. Pellets used for smoking are also food-grade. Therefore, they do not contain any adhesives or chemicals. They also don't contain softwoods, like pine or spruce, that have a high amount of sap that can adversely affect the taste of your meat.

Most wood pellets are made up of mainly oak, a very stable burning wood. This is then blended with another hardwood or fruitwood to impart the flavor through the smoke.

The Operation Principle of Traeger Wood Pellet Grill

Wood pellet grills use an auger that moves the hardwood pellets from the hopper to the fire pot underneath the grill. The higher the set temperature, the more pellets are dispensed into the auger. Once in the fire pot, a hot rod ignites the pellets creating a fire, then a fan stokes the fire creating convection heat to evenly cook your food in the grill. A drip tray sits over the fire pot, keeping the direct flames off your food while catching food drippings to help prevent flare-ups.

The Advantages of Your Traeger Wood Pellet Grill

1. The Traeger wood pellet grill makes barbecuing easy.

Plug it in, fill the hopper with BBQ pellets, turn it on, set the temperature, and let the grill do the rest. Pellet grills are designed to allow one to take a hands-off approach to cooking by letting a controller do the majority of the work.

You don't need to haul logs or arrange charcoal. You can put away the lighter fluid and flint. The Ignition sequence on a pellet grill starts with a single button press.

Once the ignition sequence is complete, the controller's capabilities determine to what extent it is able to control the cooking process. Pellet grill controllers have evolved over time from simple low, medium, & high setting devices to the advanced controllers found on high end pellet grills today.

The programs and algorithms that comprise its firmware were designed by us to ensure peak performance, consistency, and accuracy whether you're grilling steaks in the sub-zero Alaskan winter or smoking a brisket all day in the blistering deserts of Arizona.

This level of control also allows you to choose cook length, temperature, and when that temperature should change. You're in control and can fully customize the longest and most complicated of cooks to your exact specifications.

Add to this the convenience of technologies like Wi-Fi and BlueTooth and it's easy to see the appeal of the work smarter, not harder approach to smoking and grilling meat.

2. The Traeger wood pellet grill is safe.

Gas can explode. Charcoal and wood logs are messy and can smolder for days after use. Direct cooking over fire increases the likelihood of flare ups and grease fires.

Pellet grills cook indirectly, meaning no open flame, flying sparks, or direct contact between fat drippings and fire. MAK Pellet grills create small, precisely controlled fires in a stainless-steel firepot. This firepot is surrounded by a stainless-steel body and covered by a stainless-steel diffuser, and drip pan at a minimum.

Pellets are released in small quantities and consumed completely. As long as you maintain relatively minimal cleaning routines, which we make as easy as possible by using a removable firepot, the chances of anything out of the ordinary happening are extremely low.

The pellet grill is the safest outdoor cooking device ever invented.

3.Pellet grilling is better for your health and the environment. No added oils or fats are needed to achieve the tremendous flavor that cooking on a pellet grill imparts. You're cooking with real wood, which means you're using a fuel that has been used since the dawn of time. Because you are cooking indirectly, excess animal fat drippings are not burned up and made carcinogenic by open flame. Instead, they hit a grease pan and convert to gases which help flavor your food. Hardwood BBQ pellets burn with a more than 98% efficiency. This reduces the exposure of carcinogenic substances and HCA's to you and the environment. Avoiding the creation of carcinogenic smoke is not only good for your health. Extremely low particulate matter means fresher, safer air to breathe. Barbecue pellets reduce landfill disposal of sawdust by millions of tons per year. Barbecue pellets are not only a sustainable biofuel, they are also the ultimate example of re-purposing.

Tips for Using Your Traeger Wood Pellet Grill

1. Season your new pellet grill.
Season your new pellet grill according to the manufacturer's directions (a process that usually takes 45 minutes to one hour). This burns off any residual oils from the manufacturing process.

2. Allow yourself some time to get acquainted with your new grill/smoker.
Allow yourself some time to get acquainted with your new grill/smoker. We know you'll be anxious to try it out, but don't be overly ambitious. Instead of a whole brisket, which could take 15 hours or more, or a budget-busting prime rib roast, start with chicken (parts, such as breasts or wings, or a whole bird), pork loin tenderloin, or blade (shoulder) steaks, Cornish hens, salmon steaks or fillets, or other relatively inexpensive cuts that can be completed in 2 hours or less.

3. Identify any hot spots—most grills have them.
Identify any hot spots—most grills have them. Preheat your grill to medium-high as directed by the owner's manual, then lay slices of cheap white bread shoulder to shoulder across the grate. Watch carefully, then flip after a few minutes. Take a photo of the results. The darkest bread will indicate where the temperature might be hotter. (Print the photo out and add it to your owner's manual for reference.)

4. Don't let your meat come to room temperature before cooking.

Whatever meat you select, put it on the preheated grill/smoker straight from the refrigerator. Do not, as many recipes suggest, allow it to come to room temperature before cooking.

As Steven often notes, high-end steak houses do not leave their meats out at room temperature. (The danger area is 40 to 140 degrees.) The heat of the grill is sufficient to raise the internal temperature of the meat by those few degrees.

5. Invest in a good meat thermometer.

A laser-type thermometer such as this one will give you a more accurate temperature reading at grill level than a built-in dome thermometer. Determine the temperature range of your grill model from lowest to highest (180 degrees to 500+, for example).

Cleaning Your Traeger Wood Pellet Grill

For spot-cleaning the outside of your grill, you can simply use a dry cloth to remove grease marks, dust and dirt quickly. To perform a deep clean, use a soft cloth with soap and water, stainless steel cleaner or a bbq degreaser. Follow these steps to clean the outside of your BBQ:

1. Make sure your grill is cold before spraying any cleaner on the outside of your grill.
2. Apply your cleaner using a soft cloth or spray bottle. If spraying cleaner onto your pellet grill, be very careful not to get any inside of your grill. Avoid spraying stainless steel cleaner onto plastic components as it can cause them to degrade more quickly.
3. Allow the cleaner to sit for at least 30 seconds to break down any dried grease or food residue.
4. Wipe the cleaner off with a clean cloth or paper towel. If cleaning a stainless steel BBQ, wipe in the same direction as the grain. If your smoker has a painted surface, wipe in circles.
5. Repeat this process as necessary until all of the dirt and grime is removed.
6. Using a wet cloth, wipe down the surface of the grill to remove all remaining cleaner or soap residue. Do not rinse your pellet grill with a hose or bucket as water can get into the grill or hopper and cause damage its electrical components or ruin the pellets.

Always unplug your pellet grill from its power source before cleaning it with water or liquid cleaner and allow it to dry for at least 24 hours before your next grilling session. Empty your wood pellets from the hopper before cleaning and check that there is no water or cleaner in the hopper before putting the pellets back in.

SEAFOOD RECIPES

Charleston Crab Cakes With Remoulade

Servings: 4   Cooking Time: 45 Minutes

Ingredients:

- 1¼ cups mayonnaise
- ¼ cup yellow mustard
- 2 tablespoons sweet pickle relish, with its juices
- 1 tablespoon smoked paprika
- 2 teaspoons Cajun seasoning
- 2 teaspoons prepared horseradish
- 1 teaspoon hot sauce
- 1 garlic clove, finely minced
- 2 pounds fresh lump crabmeat, picked clean
- 20 butter crackers (such as Ritz brand), crushed

- 2 tablespoons Dijon mustard
- 1 cup mayonnaise
- 2 tablespoons freshly squeezed lemon juice
- 1 tablespoon salted butter, melted
- 1 tablespoon Worcestershire sauce
- 1 tablespoon Old Bay seasoning
- 2 teaspoons chopped fresh parsley
- 1 teaspoon ground mustard
- 2 eggs, beaten
- ¼ cup extra-virgin olive oil, divided

Directions:

1. For the remoulade:
2. In a small bowl, combine the mayonnaise, mustard, pickle relish, paprika, Cajun seasoning, horseradish, hot sauce, and garlic.
3. Refrigerate until ready to serve.
4. For the crab cakes:
5. Supply your smoker with wood pellets and follow the start-up procedure. Preheat, with the lid closed, to 375°F.
6. Spread the crabmeat on a foil-lined baking sheet and place over indirect heat on the grill, with the lid closed, for 30 minutes.
7. Remove from the heat and let cool for 15 minutes.
8. While the crab cools, combine the crushed crackers, Dijon mustard, mayonnaise, lemon juice, melted butter, Worcestershire sauce, Old Bay, parsley, ground mustard, and eggs until well incorporated
9. Fold in the smoked crabmeat, then shape the mixture into 8 (1-inch-thick) crab cakes.

10. In a large skillet or cast-iron pan on the grill, heat 2 tablespoons of olive oil. Add half of the crab cakes, close the lid, and smoke for 4 to 5 minutes on each side, or until crispy and golden brown.

11. Remove the crab cakes from the pan and transfer to a wire rack to drain. Pat them to remove any excess oil.

12. Repeat steps 6 and 7 with the remaining oil and crab cakes.

13. Serve the crab cakes with the remoulade.

Traeger Jerk Shrimp

Servings: 8

Cooking Time: 10 Minutes

Ingredients:

➢ 1 Tablespoon brown sugar
➢ 1 Tablespoon smoked paprika
➢ 1 Teaspoon garlic powder
➢ 1/4 Teaspoon Thyme, ground
➢ 1/4 Teaspoon ground cayenne pepper
➢ 1 Teaspoon sea salt
➢ 1 lime zest
➢ 2 Pound shrimp in shell
➢ 3 Tablespoon olive oil

Directions:

1. Combine spices, salt, and lime zest in a small bowl and mix. Place shrimp into a large bowl, then drizzle in the olive oil, Add the spice mixture and toss to combine, making sure every shrimp is kissed with deliciousness.

2. Supply your smoker with wood pellets and follow the start-up procedure. Preheat the grill, with the lid closed, to 450° F.

3. Arrange the shrimp on the grill and cook for 2 – 3 minutes per side, until firm, opaque, and cooked through. Grill: 450 °F

4. Serve with lime wedges, fresh cilantro, mint, and Caribbean Hot Pepper Sauce. Enjoy!

Cajun-blackened Shrimp

Servings: 4

Cooking Time: 20 Minutes

Ingredients:

- ➢ 1 pound peeled and deveined shrimp, with tails on
- ➢ 1 batch Cajun Rub
- ➢ 8 tablespoons (1 stick) butter
- ➢ ¼ cup Worcestershire sauce

Directions:

1. Supply your smoker with wood pellets and follow the start-up procedure. Preheat the grill, with the lid closed, to 450°F and place a cast-iron skillet on the grill grate. Wait about 10 minutes after your grill has reached temperature, allowing the skillet to get hot.

2. Meanwhile, season the shrimp all over with the rub.

3. When the skillet is hot, place the butter in it to melt. Once the butter melts, stir in the Worcestershire sauce.

4. Add the shrimp and gently stir to coat. Smoke-braise the shrimp for about 10 minutes per side, until opaque and cooked through. Remove the shrimp from the grill and serve immediately.

Grilled Maple Syrup Salmon

Servings: 6

Cooking Time: 30 Minutes

Ingredients:

➤ 1 large salmon fillet (around 3 pounds)

➤ 1/2 cup salted butter (melted)

➤ 2 tablespoons soy sauce

➤ Salt and pepper

➤ 1/4 cup maple syrup

Directions:

1. Supply your smoker with wood pellets and follow the start-up procedure. Preheat the grill, with the lid closed, to 400° F.

2. Place the salmon fillet in a baking pan lined with parchment paper.

3. Sprinkle the fish with salt and pepper.

4. Add half of the melted butter to the salmon and place the baking pan on the grill.

5. Grill for 15-20 minutes or until fish is roughly 70% cooked. It will feel still gelatinous in the thickest parts of the salmon.

6. Combine the remaining melted butter, soy sauce, and maple syrup and pour over the salmon.It will run off the sides so use a spoon to pour it back over the fish. It's also perfectly fine that some will be left on the sides of the pan.

7. Cook for 5 to 10 additional minutes or until the fish is cooked through. The fish should be firm to the touch but still moist and soft when pressed on,and the ridges will flake or pull apart if pressed on.

Pacific Northwest Salmon

Servings: 4

Cooking Time: 75 Minutes

Ingredients:

➢ 1 (2-pound) half salmon fillet

➢ 1 batch Dill Seafood Rub

➢ 2 tablespoons butter, cut into 3 or 4 slices

Directions:

1. Supply your smoker with wood pellets and follow the start-up procedure. Preheat the grill, with the lid closed, to 180°F.

2. Season the salmon all over with the rub. Using your hands, work the rub into the flesh.

3. Place the salmon directly on the grill grate, skin-side down, and smoke for 1 hour.

4. Place the butter slices on the salmon, equally spaced. Increase the grill's temperature to 300°F and continue to cook until the salmon's internal temperature reaches 145°F. Remove the salmon from the grill and serve immediately.

Flavour Fire Spiced Shrimp

Servings: 2

Cooking Time: 8 Minutes

Ingredients:

- 1 pound of extra large raw whole wild shrimp
- 1 tablespoon vegetable oil
- 1 tablespoon chili powder
- 1 teaspoon garlic powder
- 1/2 teaspoon onion powder
- 1/2 teaspoon cayenne pepper
- 1/4 teaspoon paprika
- 1/4 teaspoon dried oregano
- Pinch of Kosher salt

Directions:

1. Supply your smoker with wood pellets and follow the start-up procedure. Preheat the grill, with the lid closed, to High heat.
2. While grill is preheating, remove the shrimp shells, leaving the heads.
3. Butterfly shrimp by using a knife to cut each shrimp down the middle, from the head down to the tail.
4. Remove the vein, rinse off the shrimp and lightly dry off with paper towels.
5. Place the shrimp in a large bowl, sprinkle with all the seasonings and the oil.
6. Mix together, ensuring the mixture evenly covers each shrimp.
7. Using a skewer, impale the whole body of a shrimp, from head to tail. (Wrap them in aluminum foil if using wooden skewers).
8. Place the whole shrimp on the grill and cook for 3-4 minutes on each side (Or until shells turns pink and the shrimp is opaque).
9. Serve with your favorite sauce or condiment.

Garlic Blackened Catfish

Servings: 4

Cooking Time: 10 Minutes

Ingredients:

- ½ Cup Cajun Seasoning
- ¼ Tsp Cayenne Pepper
- 1 Tsp Granulated Garlic
- 1 Tsp Ground Thyme
- 1 Tsp Onion Powder
- 1 Tsp Ground Oregano
- 1 Tsp Pepper
- 4 (5-Oz.) Skinless Catfish Fillets
- 1 Tbsp Smoked Paprika
- 1 Stick Unsalted Butter

Directions:

1. In a small bowl, combine the Cajun seasoning, smoked paprika, onion powder, granulated garlic, ground oregano, ground thyme, pepper and cayenne pepper.

2. Sprinkle fish with salt and let rest for 20 minutes.

3. Supply your smoker with wood pellets and follow the start-up procedure. Preheat the grill, with the lid closed, to 450° F. If you're using a gas or charcoal grill, set it up for medium-high heat. Place cast iron skillet on the grill and let it preheat.

4. While grill is preheating, sprinkle catfish fillets with seasoning mixture, pressing gently to adhere. Add half the butter to preheated cast iron skillet and swirl to coat, add more butter if needed. Place fillets in hot skillet and cook 3-5 minutes or until a dark crust has been formed. Flip and cook an additional 3-5 minutes or until the fish flakes apart when pressed gently with your finger.

5. Remove fish from grill and sprinkle evenly with fresh parsley. Serve with lemon wedges and enjoy!

Lemon Scallops Wrapped In Bacon

Servings: 4

Cooking Time: 20 Minutes

Ingredients:

➢ 3 Tbsp Lemon, Juice

➢ Pepper

➢ 12 Scallop

Directions:

1. Start your grill on smoke with the lid open until a fire is established in the burn pot (3-7 minutes).

2. Supply your smoker with wood pellets and follow the start-up procedure. Preheat the grill, with the lid closed, to 400° F.Cut the bacon rashers in half, wrap each half around a scallop and use a toothpick to keep it in place.

3. Next drizzle the lemon juice over the scallops, and then place them on a baking tray.

4. Place in the grill, and grill for about 15-20 minutes, or until the bacon is crisp, remove from the grill, then serve.

Cedar Smoked Garlic Salmon

Servings: 6

Cooking Time: 60 Minutes

Ingredients:

- ➢ 1 Tsp Black Pepper
- ➢ 3 Cedar Plank, Untreated
- ➢ 1 Tsp Garlic, Minced
- ➢ 1/3 Cup Olive Oil
- ➢ 1 Tsp Onion, Salt
- ➢ 1 Tsp Parsley, Minced Fresh
- ➢ 1 1/2 Tbsp Rice Vinegar
- ➢ 2 Salmon, Fillets (Skin Removed)
- ➢ 1 Tsp Sesame Oil
- ➢ 1/3 Cup Soy Sauce

Directions:

1. Soak the cedar planks in warm water for an hour or more.
2. In a bowl, mix together the olive oil, rice vinegar, sesame oil, soy sauce, and minced garlic.
3. Add in the salmon and let it marinate for about 30 minutes.
4. Start your grill on smoke with the lid open until a fire is established in the burn pot (3-7 minutes).
5. Supply your smoker with wood pellets and follow the start-up procedure. Preheat the grill, with the lid closed, to 225° F.
6. Place the planks on the grate. Once the boards start to smoke and crackle a little, it's ready for the fish.
7. Remove the fish from the marinade, season it with the onion powder, parsley and black pepper, then discard the marinade.
8. Place the salmon on the planks and grill until it reaches 140°F internal temperature (start checking temp after the salmon has been on the grill for 30 minutes).
9. Remove from the grill, let it rest for 10 minutes, then serve.

Lemon Lobster Rolls

Servings: 4

Cooking Time: 35 Minutes

Ingredients:

- 1/2 Cup Butter
- 4 Hot Dog Bun(S)
- 1 Lemon, Whole
- 4 Lobster, Tail
- 1/4 Cup Mayo
- Pepper

Directions:

1. Supply your smoker with wood pellets and follow the start-up procedure. Preheat the grill, with the lid closed, to 300° F.

2. Using kitchen shears, cut the shell of the tail and crack in half so that the meat is exposed. Pour in butter and season with pepper. Place the tails meat side up on the grill and cook until the shell has turned red and the meat is white, about 35 minutes.

3. Remove from the grill and separate the shell from the meat. Place the meat in a bowl with mayo, lemon juice and rind and season with pepper. Stir to combine and evenly distribute into the hot dog buns.

Smoky Crab Dip

Servings: 6

Cooking Time: 20 Minutes

Ingredients:

- 1/3 Cup mayonnaise
- 3 Ounce sour cream
- 1 Teaspoon smoked paprika
- 1/4 Teaspoon cayenne pepper
- 1 1/2 Pound Crab meat, lump
- salt and pepper
- scallions, chopped
- butter crackers

Directions:

1. Supply your smoker with wood pellets and follow the start-up procedure. Preheat the grill, with the lid closed, to 350° F.

2. Meanwhile, in a large bowl gently stir together all of the ingredients except the crackers, garnish scallions and the crab meat until thoroughly combined. Gently fold in the crab meat, being careful not to break it up too much.

3. Season to taste and transfer to an oven-safe serving dish.

4. Bake for 20 to 25 minutes, until bubbly and golden on top. Grill: 350 °F

5. Garnish with the additional chopped scallions and serve warm with butter crackers. Enjoy!

Citrus-smoked Trout

Servings: 6

Cooking Time: 120 Minutes

Ingredients:

➢ 6 to 8 skin-on rainbow trout, cleaned and scaled

➢ 1 gallon orange juice

➢ ½ cup packed light brown sugar

➢ ¼ cup salt

➢ 1 tablespoon freshly ground black pepper

➢ Nonstick spray, oil, or butter, for greasing

➢ 1 tablespoon chopped fresh parsley

➢ 1 lemon, sliced

Directions:

1. Fillet the fish and pat dry with paper towels.

2. Pour the orange juice into a large container with a lid and stir in the brown sugar, salt, and pepper.

3. Place the trout in the brine, cover, and refrigerate for 1 hour.

4. Cover the grill grate with heavy-duty aluminum foil. Poke holes in the foil and spray with cooking spray (see Tip).

5. Supply your smoker with wood pellets and follow the start-up procedure. Preheat, with the lid closed, to 225°F.

6. Remove the trout from the brine and pat dry. Arrange the fish on the foil-covered grill grate, close the lid, and smoke for 1 hour 30 minutes to 2 hours, or until flaky.

7. Remove the fish from the heat. Serve garnished with the fresh parsley and lemon slices.

Grilled Salmon

Servings: 4

Cooking Time: 25 Minutes

Ingredients:

➢ 1 (2-pound) half salmon fillet

➢ 3 tablespoons mayonnaise

➢ 1 batch Dill Seafood Rub

Directions:

1. Supply your smoker with wood pellets and follow the start-up procedure. Preheat the grill, with the lid closed, to 325°F.

2. Using your hands, rub the salmon fillet all over with the mayonnaise and sprinkle it with the rub.

3. Place the salmon directly on the grill grate, skin-side down, and grill until its internal temperature reaches 145°F. Remove the salmon from the grill and serve immediately.

BAKING RECIPES

Caramel Bourbon Bacon Brownies

Servings: 16   Cooking Time: 60 Minutes

Ingredients:

- 2 Cup All-Purpose Flour
- 1/4 Cup Bourbon
- 1 Cup Brown Sugar
- 1 Cup Canola Oil
- Caramel Sauce
- 1.5 Cup Cocoa Powder
- 1 Tablespoon Hickory Honey Sea Salt
- 2 Tablespoon Instant Coffee

- 6 Large Eggs
- 1/2 Teaspoon Smoked Infused Hickory Honey Sea Salt
- 1 Cup Powdered Sugar
- 6 Slices Bacon, Raw
- 4 Tablespoons Water
- 3 Cups White Sugar

Directions:

1. Supply your smoker with wood pellets and follow the start-up procedure. Preheat the grill, with the lid closed, to 400° F.

2. In a large mixing bowl, whisk together the cocoa, powdered sugar, white sugar, instant coffee and flour.

3. To the flour mixture, add the eggs, oil and water until just combined.

4. Spray the 9 x 13 pan well with cooking spray.

5. Pour half the batter in the pan, drizzle with caramel.

6. Pour other half of batter on top and drizzle with caramel again and add candied bacon to the top.

7. Bake the brownies in the smoker for 1 hour, or until a toothpick inserted in the center of the pan comes out clean.

8. Remove from the smoker and allow to cool before slicing.

Mexican Black Bean Cornbread Casserole

Servings: 6

Cooking Time: 30 Minutes

Ingredients:

- ➢ 1 Lb Beef, Ground
- ➢ 1 15Oz Drained Black Beans, Can
- ➢ 1 Box Corn Muffin Mix
- ➢ 1 15Oz Enchilada Sauce, Can
- ➢ 1 Onion, Chopped
- ➢ 1 15Oz Drained Pinto Beans, Can

Directions:

1. Supply your smoker with wood pellets and follow the start-up procedure. Preheat the grill, with the lid closed, to 300° F.

2. Mix corn muffin mix according to directions.

3. Place cast iron skillet over flame broiler and heat for a few minutes, leaving Grill lid open.

4. Add onion and ground beef/sausage to skillet and break up

5. Cook until meat is done about 5 to 10 minutes.

6. Add both cans of beans, and enchilada sauce, stir to combine.

7. Bring mixture to a simmer.

8. Carefully close flame broiler and turn Grill up to 400 degrees.

9. Spread prepared corn muffin mix over top of meat and bean mixture and bake for 15 minutes until cornbread mixture is lightly browned.

10. Let sit 15 minutes before serving.

Savory Beaver Tails

Servings: 8

Cooking Time: 2 Minutes

Ingredients:

➢ 2 Tbsp Butter, Melted

➢ 1 Tbsp Cinnamon, Ground

➢ 1 Egg

➢ 2 1/2 Cups Flour, All-Purpose

➢ 1/2 Cup Milk, Warm

➢ 1/2 Tsp Salt

➢ 1 Tsp Sugar

➢ 1/2 Tsp Vanilla

➢ 1 L Vegetable Oil

➢ 1/4 Cup Water, Warm

➢ 2 1/2 Tsp Active Yeast, Instant

Directions:

1. In a small bowl, combine water, milk, yeast, and sugar. Let it sit for about 10 minutes or until frothy.

2. In another bowl, pour in the flour and make a well in the middle. Pour in butter, sugar, salt, vanilla and egg. Mix everything together until the dough is smooth. Knead for about 5 minutes and set the dough in a greased bowl. Cover with a towel and set aside for about an hour, or until the dough has doubled in size.

3. After one hour, supply your smoker with wood pellets and follow the start-up procedure. Preheat the grill, with the lid open, to 450° F.Pour 1L of vegetable oil into a cast iron pan and place on the grates of your Grill. Keep your flame broiler closed so as to prevent grease flareups. Preheat the oil so that it is 350 degrees F.

4. While you"re waiting for the oil to heat up, punch down the dough and separate into 8 small balls. Shape each piece of dough into a flat circle. Fry the dough in the preheated oil for about 1 minute per side, or until the dough is golden brown.

5. Sprinkle with cinnamon sugar immediately, or top with your desired toppings. Enjoy!

Cornbread Chicken Stuffing

Servings: 6 - 8

Cooking Time: 95 Minutes

Ingredients:

- 2 Tbsp Butter
- 1 Cup Chicken Stock
- 6 Cups Cornbread, Cubed
- ½ Cup Dried Cranberries
- 1 Egg
- ½ Cup Heavy Whipping Cream
- 1 Lb. Italian Sausage
- 1 Diced Onion
- 1 ½ Tsp Pulled Pork Rub
- 2 Tbsp Sage, Fresh
- ½ Tsp Fresh Thyme

Directions:

1. Supply your smoker with wood pellets and follow the start-up procedure. Preheat the grill, with the lid closed, to 250° F. If using a gas or charcoal grill, set the temp to low heat.

2. Portion sausage into quarter-size pieces and place on mesh grate. Place grate on the grill and cook for 1 hour. Sausage pieces will have a smoky deep brown color. Move the mesh tray of sausage to the side of the grill with indirect heat.

3. Open the Flame Broiler Plate and increase the temperature to 350°F. Place a large cast iron skillet on the grill, over direct flame. Add butter and onions and cook until the onions caramelize lightly, stirring often. Add the sage and thyme and stir to combine.

4. Gently fold in the dried cranberries and cubed cornbread, then add sausage directly from mesh grate.

5. In a small mixing bowl, whisk together the heavy cream, chicken stock, egg, and Pulled Pork Rub. Pour mixture over the cornbread stuffing mix.

6. Cover grill and cook 30 minutes or until heated through and crispy on top.

Smoked Blackberry Pie

Servings: 4-6

Cooking Time: 25 Minutes

Ingredients:

➤ Nonstick cooking spray or butter, for greasing

➤ 1 box (2 sheets) refrigerated piecrusts

➤ 8 tablespoons (1 stick) unsalted butter, melted, plus 8 tablespoons (1 stick) cut into pieces

➤ ½ cup all-purpose flour

➤ 2 cups sugar, divided

➤ 2 pints blackberries

➤ ½ cup milk

➤ Vanilla ice cream, for serving

Directions:

1. Supply your smoker with wood pellets and follow the start-up procedure. Preheat, with the lid closed, to 375°F.

2. Coat a cast iron skillet with cooking spray.

3. Unroll 1 refrigerated piecrust and place in the bottom and up the side of the skillet. Using a fork, poke holes in the crust in several places.

4. Set the skillet on the grill grate, close the lid, and smoke for 5 minutes, or until lightly browned. Remove from the grill and set aside.

5. In a large bowl, combine the stick of melted butter with the flour and 1½ cups of sugar.

6. Add the blackberries to the flour-sugar mixture and toss until well coated.

7. Spread the berry mixture evenly in the skillet and sprinkle the milk on top. Scatter half of the cut pieces of butter randomly over the mixture.

8. Unroll the remaining piecrust and place it over the top of skillet or slice the dough into even strips and weave it into a lattice. Scatter the remaining pieces of butter along the top of the crust.

9. Sprinkle the remaining ½ cup of sugar on top of the crust and return the skillet to the smoker.

10. Close the lid and smoke for 15 to 20 minutes, or until bubbly and brown on top. It may be necessary to use some aluminum foil around the edges near the end of the cooking time to prevent the crust from burning.

11. Serve the pie hot with vanilla ice cream.

Baked Wood-fired Pizza

Servings: 6   Cooking Time: 12 Minutes

Ingredients:

- 2/3 Cup warm water (110°F to 115°F)
- 2 1/2 Teaspoon active dry yeast
- 1/2 Teaspoon granulated sugar
- 1 Teaspoon kosher salt
- 1 Tablespoon oil
- 2 Cup all-purpose flour
- 1/4 Cup fine cornmeal
- 1 Large grilled portobello mushroom, sliced
- 1 Jar pickled artichoke hearts, drained and chopped
- 1 Cup shredded fontina cheese
- 1/2 Cup shaved Parmigiano-Reggiano cheese, divided
- To Taste Roasted Garlic, minced
- 1/4 Cup extra-virgin olive oil
- To Taste banana peppers

Directions:

1. In a glass bowl, stir together the warm water, yeast and sugar. Let stand until the mixture starts to foam, about 10 minutes. In a mixer, combine 1-3/4 cup flour, sugar and salt. Stir oil into the yeast mixture. Slowly add the liquid to the dry ingredients while slowly increasing the mixers speed until fully combined. The dough should be smooth and not sticky.

2. Knead the dough on a floured surface, gradually adding the remaining flour as needed to prevent the dough from sticking, until smooth, about 5 to 10 minutes.

3. Form the dough into a ball. Apply a thin layer of olive oil to a large bowl. Place the dough into the bowl and coat the dough ball with a small amount of olive oil. Cover and let rise in a warm place for about 1 hour or until doubled in size.

4. When ready to cook, set smoker temperature to 450°F and preheat, lid closed for 15 minutes.

5. Place a pizza stone in the grill while it preheats.

6. Punch the dough down and roll it out into a 12-inch circle on a floured surface.

7. Spread the cornmeal evenly on the pizza peel. Place the dough on the pizza peel and assemble the toppings evenly in the following order: olive oil, roasted garlic, fontina, portobello, artichoke hearts, Parmigiano-Reggiano and banana peppers.

8. Carefully slide the assembled pizza from the pizza peel to the preheated pizza stone and bake until the crust is golden brown, about 10 to 12 minutes. Enjoy!

Smoker Wheat Bread

Servings: 6   Cooking Time: 60 Minutes

Ingredients:

- As Needed extra-virgin olive oil
- 2 Cup all-purpose flour
- 1 Cup whole wheat flour
- 1 1/4 Ounce Packet, Active Dry Yeast
- 1 1/4 Teaspoon salt
- 1 1/2 Cup water
- As Needed Cornmeal

Directions:

1. Oil a large mixing bowl and set aside. In a second mixing bowl, combine the flours, yeast, and salt.
2. Push your sleeve up to your elbow and form your fingers into a claw. Mix the dry ingredients until well-combined.
3. Add the water and mix until blended. The dough will be wet, shaggy, and somewhat stringy.
4. Tip the dough into the oiled mixing bowl and cover with plastic wrap.
5. Allow the dough to rise at room temperature-- about 70 degrees-- for 2 hours, or until the surface is bubbled.
6. Turn the dough out onto a lightly floured work surface and lightly flour the top. With floured hands, fold the dough over on itself twice. Cover loosely with plastic wrap and allow the dough to rest for 15 minutes.
7. Dust a clean lint-free cotton towel with cornmeal, wheat bran, or flour. With floured hands, gently form the dough into a ball and place it, seam side down, on the towel.
8. Dust the top of the ball with cornmeal, wheat bran, or flour, and cover the dough with a second towel. Let the dough rise until doubled in size; the dough will not spring back when poked with a finger.
9. In the meantime, start the smoker grill and set temperature to 450 F. Preheat, lid closed, for 10-15 minutes.
10. Put a lidded 6- to 8-quart cast iron Dutch oven - preferably one coated with enamel, on the grill grate.
11. When the dough has risen, remove the top towel, slide your hand under the bottom towel to support the dough, then carefully tip the dough, seam side up, into the preheated pot.
12. Remove the towel. Shake the pot a couple of times if the dough looks lopsided: It will straighten out as it bakes.
13. Cover the pot with the lid and bake the bread for 30 minutes. Remove the lid and continue to bake the bread for 15 to 30 minutes more, or until it is nicely browned and sounds hollow when rapped with your knuckles.
14. Turn onto a wire rack to cool. Slice with a serrated knife. Enjoy!

Baked Buttermilk Biscuits

Servings: 4

Cooking Time: 15 Minutes

Ingredients:

➢ 2 Cup all-purpose flour

➢ 1/4 Cup butter

➢ 3/4 Cup buttermilk

Directions:

1. Supply your smoker with wood pellets and follow the start-up procedure. Preheat the grill, with the lid closed, to High heat. Spoon the flour into a measuring cup and level with a knife.

2. Put the flour into a mixing bowl. Using a pastry blender, cut the butter into the flour until the mixture resembles coarse crumbs.

3. With a fork, gently stir in just enough of the buttermilk so the dough leaves the sides of the bowl. (You may not need all the buttermilk.) For the most tender biscuits, do not overmix.

4. Lightly flour a work surface as well as your hands. Tip the dough onto the floured surface and gently bring together using your fingertips. (Re-flour your hands or the board if the dough is too sticky.) Knead two or three times, just to bring the dough together.

5. With a floured rolling pin, lightly and quickly roll the dough out to a thickness of about 1/2". Using a 1-1/2" floured cutter, cut out as many biscuits as you can. (Do not twist the cutter; push it straight down.) You can reroll the scraps if desired, but the "second string" biscuits will be tougher.

6. Transfer the biscuits to an ungreased baking sheet. Using a pastry brush, brush the tops with melted butter. Bake until golden brown, 10 to 15 minutes. Enjoy! Grill: 500 °F

Smoky Apple Crepes

Servings: 6   Cooking Time: 60 Minutes

Ingredients:

- 1/2 Cup Apple Juice
- 2 Lbs Apples
- 2 Tbsp Brown Sugar
- 5 Tbsp Butter
- 3 Tbsp Butter, Melted
- Tt Caramel
- 3/4 Tsp Cinnamon, Ground
- Tt Cinnamon-Sugar
- 3/4 Tsp Cornstarch
- 2 Eggs
- 1 Cup Flour
- 2 Tsp Lemon Juice
- Tennessee Apple Butter Seasoning
- 1/2 Cup Water
- 3/4 Cup Milk

Directions:

1. Supply your smoker with wood pellets and follow the start-up procedure. Preheat the grill, with the lid closed, to 225° F. If using a gas or charcoal grill, set it up for low, indirect heat.

2. Peel, halve, and core apples.

3. Season apples with Tennessee Apple Butter then place directly on the grill grate, and smoke for 1 hour.

4. Meanwhile, prepare crêpe batter: combine eggs, milk, water, flour, and 3 tbsp of melted butter in a blender, and blend until smooth.

5. Refrigerate for 30 minutes.

6. Remove apples from grill, cool slightly, then slice thin.

7. Place a cast iron skillet on the grill and melt 3 tbsp butter with brown sugar, cinnamon, cornstarch, apple and lemon juices. Cook for 5 minutes until thick.

8. Add apples and cook for another 3 to 5 minutes, stirring to coat apples in sauce.

9. Remove from grill and set aside.

10. Preheat griddle to medium-low. If using a standard grill, preheat a cast iron skillet on medium-low heat.

11. Melt 1 teaspoon of butter on the griddle.

12. Then add ½ cup of batter, and spread with the bottom of a metal spatula, working quickly, as the batter cooks fast.

13. Cook one minute per side, until edges begin to brown. Remove from griddle, set aside, and repeat with remaining batter.

14. Spoon ¼ cup of apple filling into the center of each crêpe, then quarter-fold into a triangle.

15. Serve warm with additional apple filling, drizzle of warm caramel, and a dusting of cinnamon-sugar.

Baked Peach Cobbler Cupcakes

Servings: 8

Cooking Time: 30 Minutes

Ingredients:

- 2 Large Peaches, fresh
- 3/4 Cup sugar
- 2 Teaspoon lemon juice
- 1/2 Teaspoon ground cinnamon
- Yellow Cake Mix, Boxed
- 1 Can vanilla icing

Directions:

1. Bring a pot of water to a boil. Turn peaches upside down and cut a small shallow X across the bottom. Put peaches in boiling water and boil for 1 minute to help loosen the skin.

2. Drain the peaches into a colander and rinse off with cold water. Peel skin off peaches.

3. Filling: Dice peaches and place into a large pan. Cook peaches over medium heat. As it starts to sizzle, add sugar, lemon and cinnamon. Cook mixture on medium heat for 10-15 minutes until a majority of the juice from the peaches evaporates leaving a thick syrup.

4. Transfer to a bowl to cool.

5. Supply your smoker with wood pellets and follow the start-up procedure. Preheat the grill, with the lid closed, to 350° F.

6. Cupcakes: Follow the directions on box cake mix and put the mixture into cupcake pan with liners.

7. When grill has preheated, bake cupcakes for 13-16 minutes, until a light golden brown. Grill: 350 °F

8. When cupcakes have cooled, use a piping bag to pipe the peach cobbler mixture into the middle of the cupcake.

9. Ice with your favorite vanilla icing. Enjoy!

Grilled Apple Pie

Servings: 4

Cooking Time: 40 Minutes

Ingredients:

- ➤ 5 Whole Apples
- ➤ 1/4 Cup sugar
- ➤ 1 Tablespoon cornstarch
- ➤ 1 Whole refrigerated pie crust
- ➤ 1/4 Cup Peach, preserves

Directions:

1. Supply your smoker with wood pellets and follow the start-up procedure. Preheat the grill, with the lid closed, to 375° F.In a medium bowl, mix the apples, sugar, and cornstarch; set aside.

2. Unroll pie crust. Place in ungreased pie pan. With the back of a spoon, spread preserves evenly on crust. Arrange the apple slices in an even layer in the pie pan. Slightly fold crust over filling.

3. Place a baking sheet upside down on the grill grate to make an elevated surface. Put the pan with pie on top so it is elevated off grill. (This will help prevent the bottom from overcooking.) Cook the pie for 30 to 40 minutes or until crust is golden brown, the filling is bubbly. Grill: 375 °F

4. Remove from grill; cool 10 minutes before serving. Enjoy! *Cook times will vary depending on set and ambient temperatures.

Vanilla Chocolate Bacon Cupcakes

Servings: 12

Cooking Time: 120 Minutes

Ingredients:

- 1 Lb Bacon
- 1 1/2 Tsp Baking Powder
- 1 1/2 Tsp Baking Soda
- 1 Cup Cocoa, Powder
- 2 Egg
- 1 3/4 Cups Flour
- 1 Cup Milk, Whole
- 1/2 Cup Oil
- 1 Tsp Salt
- 2 Cups Sugar
- 2 Tsp Vanilla

Directions:

1. Supply your smoker with wood pellets and follow the start-up procedure. Preheat the grill, with the lid closed, to 250° F.

2. Once your grill is preheated, place bacon strips on the grates. Smoke for 1hr-1 ½ hours or until desired crispiness is achieved.

3. Remove the bacon from the grill and set aside.

4. Increase set the temperature to 350°F and preheat.

5. Mix the rest of the ingredients in a bowl with an electric mixer until it is nice and smooth.

6. Pour the mixture into a cupcake tin.

7. Transfer the tin to your grill and bake for about 20 - 25 minutes.

8. Allow the cupcakes to cool on a wire rack. Once cooled, top with your favorite premade icing and a half of strip of the bacon. Serve and enjoy!

Onion Cheese Nachos

Servings: 6

Cooking Time: 10 Minutes

Ingredients:

➢ 1 Pound Beef, Ground

➢ 3 Cups Cheddar Cheese, Shredded

➢ 1 Green Bell Pepper, Diced

➢ 1/2 Cup Green Onion

➢ 1/2 Cup Red Onion, Diced

➢ 1 Large Bag Tortilla Chip

Directions:

1. Supply your smoker with wood pellets and follow the start-up procedure. Preheat the grill, with the lid closed, to 350° F.

2. While you're waiting, empty a large bag of nacho chips evenly onto a cast iron pan. Start loading up with toppings - cooked ground beef, red onion, red pepper, cheese, green onions. These are just the toppings we had on hand, so feel free to add anything you like! Make sure you do a couple layers of chips so everyone gets a good serving of nachos. And don't be skimpy with the cheese - lay it on heavy!

3. Place your loaded nachos on the grill and let the hot smoke melt your toppings into one cheesy creation. Heat at 350°F for 10 minutes or until the cheese has fully melted. Remove and serve with sour-cream and salsa.

PORK RECIPES

Grilled Pork Tacos Al Pastor

Servings: 8   Cooking Time: 15 Minutes

Ingredients:

- 2 Tsp Annatto Powder
- Cilantro, Chopped
- Corn Tortillas
- 2 Tsp Cumin
- 1 Tsp Granulated Garlic
- 2 Tbsp Guajillo Chili Powder
- Jalapeno Pepper, Minced
- Lime, Wedges
- 1 Tsp Oregano, Dried
- 1/2 Tsp Pepper
- 1/2 Cup Pineapple, Juice
- 1/2 Pineapple, Skinned & Cored
- 2 Lbs Pork Shoulder, Boneless, Sliced Thin
- 1 1/2 Tsp Salt
- 2 Tbsp Tomato Paste
- 2 Tbsp Vegetable Oil
- 1/4 Cup White Vinegar
- Yellow Onion, Chopped

Directions:

1. Prepare marinade: In a mixing bowl, whisk together pineapple juice, vinegar, oil, tomato paste, chili powder, annatto, cumin, granulated garlic, oregano, salt, and pepper. Set aside.

2. Slice pork shoulder into thin slices (around ¼" thick), then place in a resealable plastic bag. Pour marinade over pork, seal bag, and turn to coat. Refrigerate overnight.

3. Supply your smoker with wood pellets and follow the start-up procedure. Preheat the grill, with the lid open, to 450° F. If using a gas or charcoal grill, set it up for high heat.

4. Remove the pork from the marinade and set on the grill. Grill over high heat for 3 to 5 minutes, turning frequently. Transfer to a cutting board to rest for 10 minutes, then slice thin.

5. Grill pineapple for 3 minutes, turning once. Set aside on a cutting board, and chop once cooled.

6. Assemble tacos: tortillas, pork, pineapple, jalapeño, onion, and cilantro. Serve warm with fresh lime wedges.

Pork Belly Burnt Ends

Servings: 8-10

Cooking Time: 360 Minutes

Ingredients:

➢ 1 (3-pound) skinless pork belly (if not already skinned, use a sharp boning knife to remove the skin from the belly), cut into 1½- to 2-inch cubes

➢ 1 batch Sweet Brown Sugar Rub

➢ ½ cup honey

➢ 1 cup The Ultimate BBQ Sauce

➢ 2 tablespoons light brown sugar

Directions:

1. Supply your smoker with wood pellets and follow the start-up procedure. Preheat the grill, with the lid closed, to 250°F.

2. Generously season the pork belly cubes with the rub. Using your hands, work the rub into the meat.

3. Place the pork cubes directly on the grill grate and smoke until their internal temperature reaches 195°F.

4. Transfer the cubes from the grill to an aluminum pan. Add the honey, barbecue sauce, and brown sugar. Stir to combine and coat the pork.

5. Place the pan in the grill and smoke the pork for 1 hour, uncovered. Remove the pork from the grill and serve immediately.

Sweet Bacon

Servings: 4

Cooking Time: 60 Minutes

Ingredients:
- 1 Pack Bacon, Thick Cut
- 1/2 Cup Brown Sugar
- 1/2 Cup Maple Syrup
- Mandarin Habanero Seasoning

Directions:

1. Place the bacon in a deep dish. Add the maple syrup, cover and refrigerate 2 - 3 hours or overnight.

2. Supply your smoker with wood pellets and follow the start-up procedure. Preheat the grill, with the lid open, to 225° F.

3. When the grill has preheated, place the bacon directly on the cooking grids and sprinkle with brown sugar and Mandarin Habanero. Check every 15-20. After 30 minutes, flip and rotate bacon and baste with syrup. Allow to hot smoke for another 20 to 30 minutes or until the bacon is done to your desired liking.

4. Allow to cool on a rack and serve.

5. Can be refrigerated in an airtight container.

Stuffed Pork Crown Roast

Servings: 2-4   Cooking Time: 180 Minutes

Ingredients:

- 10 Pound Crown Roast of Pork, 12-14 ribs
- 1 Cup apple juice or cider
- 2 Tablespoon apple cider vinegar
- 2 Tablespoon Dijon mustard
- 1 Tablespoon brown sugar
- 2 Clove garlic, minced
- 2 Tablespoon Thyme or Rosemary, fresh

- 1 Teaspoon salt
- 1 Teaspoon coarse ground black pepper, divided
- 1/2 Cup olive oil
- 8 Cup Your Favorite Stuffing, Prepared According to the Package Directions, or Homemade

Directions:

1. Set the pork on a flat rack in a shallow roasting pan. Cover the end of each bone with a small piece of foil.

2. Make the marinade: Bring the apple cider to a boil over high heat and reduce by half. Remove from the heat, and whisk in the vinegar, mustard, brown sugar, garlic, thyme, and salt and pepper. Slowly whisk in the oil.

3. Using a pastry brush, apply the marinade to the roast, coating all surfaces. Cover it with plastic wrap and allow it to sit until the meat comes to room temperature, about 1 hour.

4. When ready to cook, set grill temperature to High and preheat, lid closed for 15 minutes.

5. Arrange the roasting pan with the pork on the grill grate. Roast for 30 minutes.

6. Reduce the heat to 325℉. Loosely fill the crown with the stuffing, mounding it at the top. Cover the stuffing with foil. (Alternatively, you can bake the stuffing in a separate pan alongside the roast.)

7. Roast the pork for another 1-1/2 hours. Remove the foil from the stuffing and continue to roast until the internal temperature of the meat is 150℉, about 30 minutes to an hour. Make sure the temperature probe doesn't touch bone or you will get a false reading.

8. Remove roast from grill and allow to rest for 15 minutes. Remove the foil covering the bones, but leave the butcher's string on the roast until ready to carve. Transfer to a warm platter.

9. To serve, carve between the bones. Enjoy!

Scalloped Potatoes With Ham, Corn And Bacon

Servings: 4-6

Cooking Time: 60 Minutes

Ingredients:

- ➤ 1 1/2 Cups Cooked Bacon, Chopped
- ➤ 1 Tablespoon Butter
- ➤ 1 1/2 Cup Cooked Ham, Cubed
- ➤ 5-6 Large Potatoes, Red
- ➤ Salt And Pepper
- ➤ 1 Cup Whole Kernel Corn
- ➤ Milk

Directions:

1. Supply your smoker with wood pellets and follow the start-up procedure. Preheat the grill, with the lid open, to 350° F.

2. Smear softened butter all over the bottom of a baking dish. Slice potatoes as uniformly as possible.

3. Place enough potatoes in the pan to cover the bottom. Add some of the bacon, ham and corn on top of the potatoes. Repeat this until you've created a few layers and have used all the potatoes, ham, corn and bacon.

4. Add 1 tbsp of butter and cover with milk, till it's almost covering the mixture. Add salt and pepper to taste.

5. Place on the grill for 1 hour and enjoy!

Beer Pork Belly Chili Con Carne

Servings: 4   Cooking Time: 120 Minutes

Ingredients:

- Avocado, Diced
- 2 Bay Leaves
- 1 Lbs Beef Stew Meat
- 12 Oz Beef Stock
- 12 Oz Beer, Bottle
- 15 Oz Black Beans, Rinsed And Drained
- 3 Tbsp Chili Powder
- Cilantro, Chopped
- 1 Tsp Coriander, Ground
- 2 Tsp Cumin, Ground
- 1 Tbsp Flour
- 4 Garlic Cloves, Minced
- 2 Tsp Mexican Oregano, Dried
- 2 Tbsp Olive Oil
- 2 Oz Pancetta, Diced
- Pork Belly, Cut Into 1 Inch Chunks
- 2 Red Onion, Chopped
- Rice, Cooked
- To Taste, Salt & Pepper
- Scallion, Sliced Thin
- 1/4 Cup Tomato Purée

Directions:

1. Supply your smoker with wood pellets and follow the start-up procedure. Preheat the grill, with the lid open, to 425° F. If using a gas or charcoal grill, set it up for medium-high heat. Place Dutch oven on grill and allow to preheat.

2. Heat the olive oil in the Dutch oven, then sauté the pancetta until crisp. Add the onions and sauté for 3 minutes, then add the garlic and sauté 1 minute, until fragrant. Remove mixture with a slotted spoon and set aside.

3. Add the pork belly and beef to the pot to brown, then add the chili powder, cumin, oregano, and coriander. Add the flour and cook for 2 minutes, stirring constantly.

4. Add the beer, beef stock, and tomato purée. Stir well, then return the pancetta mixture to the pot. Add the black beans and bay leaves, then season with salt and pepper.

5. Bring chili to a simmer, then reduce temperature to 325°F and simmer, uncovered, for 2 hours, stirring occasionally, until meat is tender, and sauce has thickened.

6. Remove the chili from the grill, then serve warm with cooked rice, avocado, fresh cilantro, and scallions.

Smoked Bbq Ribs

Servings: 4

Cooking Time: 300 Minutes

Ingredients:

➢ 2 Rack St. Louis-style ribs

➢ 1/4 Cup Big Game Rub

➢ 1 Cup apple juice

➢ BBQ Sauce

Directions:

1. Pat ribs dry and peel the membrane from the back of the ribs.

2. Apply an even coat of rub to the front, back and sides of the ribs. Let sit for 20 minutes and up to 4 hours if refrigerated.

3. Supply your smoker with wood pellets and follow the start-up procedure. Preheat the grill, with the lid closed, to 225° F.

4. Place ribs, bone side down on grill. Put apple juice in a spray bottle and spray the ribs after 1 hour of cooking. Spray every 45 minutes thereafter. Grill: 225 °F Probe: 201 °F

5. After 4-1/2 hours, check the internal temperature of ribs. Ribs are done when internal temperature reaches 201°F. If not, check back in another 30 minutes. Grill: 225 °F Probe: 201 °F

6. Once ribs are done, brush a light layer of your favorite Traeger BBQ Sauce on the front and back of the ribs. Let the sauce set for 10 minutes. After the sauce has set, take ribs off the grill and let rest for 10 minutes. Slice ribs in between the bones and serve with extra sauce. Enjoy!

Whiskey- & Cider-brined Pork Shoulder

Servings: 8   Cooking Time: 540 Minutes

Ingredients:

- 1 bone-in pork shoulder, about 5 to 7lb (2.3 to 3.2kg)
- fresh coarsely ground black pepper
- granulated garlic
- 1 cup apple juice or apple cider
- low-carb barbecue sauce, warmed
- hamburger buns (optional)

- for the brine
- 1 gallon (3.8 liters) cold distilled water
- 1 cup coarse salt
- 1¼ cup whiskey, divided
- ½ cup light brown sugar or low-carb substitute

Directions:

1. In a large saucepot on the stovetop over medium-high heat, make the brine by bringing the water, salt, 1 cup of whiskey, and brown sugar to a boil. Stir with a long-handled wooden spoon until the salt and sugar dissolve. Let the brine cool to room temperature. Cover and cool completely in the refrigerator.

2. Submerge the pork in the brine. If it floats, place a resealable bag of ice on top. Refrigerate for 24 hours.

3. Supply your smoker with wood pellets and follow the start-up procedure. Preheat the grill, with the lid closed, to 250° F.

4. Remove the pork shoulder from the brine and pat dry with paper towels. (Discard the brine.) Season the pork with pepper and granulated garlic. Place the pork on the grate and smoke until the internal temperature reaches 165°F (74°C), about 5 hours.

5. Transfer the pork to an aluminum foil roasting pan and add the apple juice and the remaining ¼ cup of whiskey. Cover tightly with aluminum foil. Place the pan on the grate and cook the pork until the bone releases easily from the meat and the internal temperature reaches 200°F (93°C), about 3 hours more. (Be careful when lifting a corner of the foil to check on the roast because steam will escape.)

6. Remove the pan from the grill and let the pork rest for 20 minutes. Reserve the juices.

7. Wearing heatproof gloves, pull the pork into chunks. Discard the bone or any large lumps of fat. Pull the meat into shreds and transfer to a clean aluminum foil roasting pan. Moisten with the barbecue sauce or serve the sauce on the side. Stir in some of the drippings—not too much because you don't want the pork to be swimming in its juices. Serve on buns (if using).

Bbq Pulled Pork With Sweet & Heat Bbq Sauce

Servings: 4

Cooking Time: 540 Minutes

Ingredients:

- ➢ 10 Pound Bone-In Pork Butt
- ➢ 2 Tablespoon Pork & Poultry Rub
- ➢ 1 1/2 Cup apple juice
- ➢ 4 Tablespoon brown sugar
- ➢ 1 Tablespoon salt
- ➢ 1 To Taste salt
- ➢ 1 To Taste Pork & Poultry Rub
- ➢ 1 As Needed Sweet & Heat BBQ Sauce

Directions:

1. Trim pork butt of all excess fat leaving 1/4" of the fat cap attached. Combine 2 Tbsp Pork and Poultry rub, apple juice, brown sugar, and salt in a small bowl stirring until most of the sugar and salt are dissolved. Inject the pork butt every square inch or so with the apple juice mixture. Season the exterior of the pork butt with remaining rub.

2. Supply your smoker with wood pellets and follow the start-up procedure. Preheat the grill, with the lid closed, to 225° F.

3. Place pork butt directly on the grill grate and cook for about 6 hours or until the internal temperature reaches 160°F. Grill: 225 °F Probe: 160 °F

4. Wrap the pork butt in two layers of foil and pour in 1/2 cup of apple juice. Secure tin foil tightly to contain the apple juice. Increase temperature to 275°F and return to grill in a pan large enough to hold the pork butt in case of leaks. Cook an additional 3 hours or until internal temperature reaches 205°F. Grill: 275 °F Probe: 205 °F

5. Remove from the grill and discard the bone. Shred the pork removing any excess fat or tendons. Season with additional Pork and Poultry Rub and salt if needed.

6. Add Sweet & Heat BBQ sauce and serve. Enjoy!

3-2-1 Bbq Baby Back Ribs

Servings: 6   Cooking Time: 360 Minutes

Ingredients:

- 2 Rack baby back pork ribs
- 1/3 Cup yellow mustard
- 1/2 Cup apple juice, divided
- 1 Tablespoon Worcestershire sauce

- Pork & Poultry Rub
- 1/2 Cup dark brown sugar
- 1/3 Cup honey, warmed
- 1 Cup 'Que BBQ Sauce

Directions:

1. If your butcher has not already done so, remove the thin silverskin membrane from the bone-side of the ribs by working the tip of a butter knife or a screwdriver underneath the membrane over a middle bone. Use paper towels to get a firm grip, then tear the membrane off.

2. In a small bowl, combine the mustard, 1/4 cup of apple juice (reserve the rest) and the Worcestershire sauce. Spread the mixture thinly on both sides of the ribs and season with Traeger Pork & Poultry Rub.

3. Supply your smoker with wood pellets and follow the start-up procedure. Preheat the grill, with the lid closed, to 180° F.Smoke the ribs, meat-side up for 3 hours.

4. After the ribs have smoked for 3 hours, transfer them to a rimmed baking sheet and increase the grill temperature to 225°F.

5. Tear off four long sheets of heavy-duty aluminum foil. Top with a rack of ribs and pull up the sides to keep the liquid enclosed. Sprinkle half the brown sugar on the rack, then top with half the honey and half the remaining apple juice. Use a bit more apple juice if you want more tender ribs. Lay another piece of foil on top and tightly crimp the edges so there is no leakage. Repeat with the remaining rack of ribs.

6. Return the foiled ribs to the grill and cook for an additional 2 hours.

7. Carefully remove the foil from the ribs and brush the ribs on both sides with Traeger 'Que Sauce. Discard the foil. Arrange the ribs directly on the grill grate and continue to grill until the sauce tightens, 30 to 60 minutes more.

8. Let the ribs rest for a few minutes before serving. Enjoy!

The Dan Patrick Show Baked Chili Cheese Dog Cups

Servings: 6

Cooking Time: 30 Minutes

Ingredients:

➢ 2 Cup Chili With Beans, Your Choice

➢ 2 Olympia Provisions Franks

➢ 1 Can Pillsbury Grands Buttermilk Biscuits

Directions:

1. Supply your smoker with wood pellets and follow the start-up procedure. Preheat the grill, with the lid closed, to 350° F.

2. Combine chili and sliced hot dogs in a medium bowl. Open biscuits and separate into 8 biscuits.

3. Place each biscuit in a lightly greased muffin tin and press down on the sides and bottom to create a cup. Spoon a little bit of the chili hot dog mixture into each cup.

4. Place muffin tin directly on the grill grate and cook 30 minutes until biscuits are golden brown and chili is warmed. Grill: 350 ˚F

5. Let chili cups cool for five minutes before unmolding. Finish with your choice of toppings. Enjoy!

Pulled Pork Corn Tortillas

Servings: 4

Cooking Time: 15 Minutes

Ingredients:

➢ Cilantro

➢ Cilantro, Chopped

➢ 8 Corn Tortillas

➢ Jalepeno, Sliced

➢ 1 Lime, Wedges

➢ 2 Cups Pulled Pork

➢ Radishes, Sliced

➢ White Onion, Diced

Directions:

1. Supply your smoker with wood pellets and follow the start-up procedure. Preheat the grill, with the lid open, to 350° F. Grill the corn tortillas until they are softened and have charred spots, about 30 seconds.

2. To assemble the carnitas, add the pulled pork to the tortillas, and top with radishes, diced onion, cilantro, jalapeno and a squeeze of lime juice, if desired. Serve and enjoy!

Smoked Stuffed Avocado Recipe

Servings: 8

Cooking Time: 30 Minutes

Ingredients:

- ➢ 6 Whole avocados
- ➢ 3 Cup leftover pulled pork
- ➢ 1 1/2 Cup Monterey Jack cheese, shredded
- ➢ 1 Cup Salsa, tomato
- ➢ 1/4 Cup cilantro, finely chopped
- ➢ 8 Whole Quail Eggs

Directions:

1. Supply your smoker with wood pellets and follow the start-up procedure. Preheat the grill, with the lid closed, to 375° F.

2. Remove the pits from the avocados, removing some avocado from the center if needed.

3. In a bowl, mix together pork, cheese, salsa and cilantro. Place pork mixture on top of avocados and place in grill. Cook for 25 minutes.

4. Take a spoon and make a divot or "nest" for the quail egg. Carefully crack the quail egg into the "nest" and cook for an additional 5 to 8 minutes or until the egg reaches desired doneness.

5. Remove from the grill and serve. Enjoy!

VEGETABLES RECIPES

Traeger Smoked Coleslaw

Servings: 8

Cooking Time: 20 Minutes

Ingredients:

➢ 1 Head purple cabbage, shredded

➢ 1 Head green cabbage, shredded

➢ 1 Cup shredded carrots

➢ 2 scallions, thinly sliced

➢ 1 1/2 Cup mayonnaise

➢ 1/8 Cup white wine vinegar

➢ 1 Teaspoon celery seed

➢ 1 Teaspoon sugar

➢ salt and pepper

Directions:

1. Supply your smoker with wood pellets and follow the start-up procedure. Preheat the grill, with the lid closed, to 180° F.

2. Spread cabbage and carrots out on a sheet tray and place directly on the grill grates. Smoke for 20 to 25 minutes or until cabbage picks up desired amount of smoke. Grill: 180 °F

3. Remove from grill and transfer to the refrigerator immediately to cool. While cabbage is cooling, make the dressing.

4. For the dressing, combine all ingredients in a small bowl and mix well.

5. Place smoked cabbage and carrots in a large bowl and pour dressing over them. Stir to coat well.

6. Transfer to a serving dish and sprinkle with scallions. Enjoy!

Roasted New Potatoes

Servings: 4

Cooking Time: 25 Minutes

Ingredients:

➤ 2 Pound small new potatoes

➤ 3 Tablespoon butter, melted

➤ 2 Tablespoon olive oil

➤ 2 Tablespoon whole mustard seeds

➤ salt and pepper

➤ 2 Tablespoon freshly minced chives

➤ 2 Tablespoon freshly minced parsley

Directions:

1. Place potatoes in a colander and rinse with cold water. Dry on paper towels and transfer to a rimmed baking sheet large enough to hold them in a single layer.

2. Drizzle the potatoes with butter and olive oil, then sprinkle them with the mustard seeds. Season with salt and pepper.

3. Supply your smoker with wood pellets and follow the start-up procedure. Preheat the grill, with the lid closed, to 400° F.

4. Place the baking sheet with the potatoes on the grill grate. Roast for about 25 minutes shaking the pan once or twice, until potatoes are tender and the skins are slightly wrinkled. Grill: 400 °F

5. Transfer potatoes to a bowl or platter. Top with fresh chives and parsley. Enjoy!

Stuffed Jalapenos

Servings: 8

Cooking Time: 60 Minutes

Ingredients:

➤ 40 Whole jalapeño

➤ 8 Ounce cream cheese, room temperature

➤ 1 Cup Sharp Cheddar Grated

➤ 1 1/2 Teaspoon Pork & Poultry Rub

➤ 2 Tablespoon sour cream

➤ 1 Whole (14 oz) cocktail sausages

➤ 20 Whole Slices of Smoked Bacon, Cut in Half

Directions:

1. Wash and dry the peppers. Cut the stem ends off with a paring knife, and using the same knife or a small metal spoon, carefully scrape the seeds and ribs out of each pepper. Set aside.

2. In a small bowl, combine the cream cheese, grated cheese, Traeger Pork and Poultry Rub, and the sour cream.

3. Transfer the mixture to a sturdy resealable plastic bag and trim 1/2-inch off one of the lower corners with a scissors. Squeeze the cream cheese mixture into each pepper, filling each a little over the halfway point.

4. Stuff one sausage into each pepper. Wrap the outside of each with a piece of bacon, securing with 1 or 2 toothpicks.

5. Arrange the peppers on a foil-lined baking sheet. Supply your smoker with wood pellets and follow the start-up procedure. Preheat the grill, with the lid closed, to 180° F, and smoke the peppers for 1 to 1-1/2 hours.

6. Increase the heat to 350 degrees F and continue to cook for 20 to 30 minutes, or until the bacon begins to render its fat and crisp. Enjoy! Grill: 350 °F

Red Potato Grilled Lollipops

Servings: 4

Cooking Time: 25 Minutes

Ingredients:

- ➢ 8 Large red bliss potatoes, halved
- ➢ 2 Clove garlic, minced
- ➢ 2 Sprig rosemary, minced
- ➢ 2 Tablespoon olive oil
- ➢ 1 Teaspoon salt
- ➢ 1/2 Teaspoon black pepper
- ➢ 5 Wooden Skewers, soaked in water
- ➢ 1/4 Cup Parmesan cheese, grated

Directions:

1. Supply your smoker with wood pellets and follow the start-up procedure. Preheat the grill, with the lid closed, to 450° F.

2. Halve potatoes and poke each several times with a fork.

3. Put the potatoes in a large bowl and toss with the minced garlic, rosemary leaves, a few tablespoons of olive oil, kosher salt, and pepper. Microwave the potatoes for 4 minutes. Gently toss potatoes and microwave for another 3 minutes.

4. Skewer potato halves threading about 4 or 5 potato halves on each skewer. Brush potatoes with olive oil.

5. Place the potato skewers on the Traeger, cut side down, and grill until the sides begin to brown (4-7 minutes).

6. Flip and grill skin side down for another 7-10 minutes.

7. They are done when a sharp knife tip easily penetrates the sides. Remove potatoes from grill and top with grated parmesan cheese. Enjoy!

Grilled Asparagus And Spinach Salad

Servings: 8

Cooking Time: 10 Minutes

Ingredients:

➢ 4 Fluid Ounce apple cider vinegar

➢ 8 Fluid Ounce Honey Bourbon BBQ Sauce

➢ 2 Bunch asparagus, ends trimmed

➢ 3 Fluid Ounce extra-virgin olive oil

➢ 2 Ounce Beef Rub

➢ 24 Ounce Spinach, fresh

➢ 4 Ounce candied pecans

➢ 4 Ounce feta cheese

Directions:

1. Combine apple cider vinegar and Traeger Apricot BBQ Sauce to create salad dressing.

2. Supply your smoker with wood pellets and follow the start-up procedure. Preheat the grill, with the lid closed, to High heat.

3. Toss the asparagus with Olive Oil and the Beef Shake. Put asparagus in the Traeger Grilling Basket and move the basket to the grill grate.

4. Grill for about 10 minutes. Remove the asparagus once it is cooked. Grill: 350 °F

5. Place the hot asparagus right on top of the bowl of spinach.

6. Add candied pecans, feta cheese & salad dressing then toss and serve. Enjoy!

Bacon Wrapped Corn On The Cob

Servings: 4

Cooking Time: 21 Minutes

Ingredients:

➢ 4 Whole Corn, ears

➢ 8 Slices bacon

➢ 1 Teaspoon freshly ground black pepper

➢ 1 Teaspoon chili powder

➢ 1 To Taste Parmesan cheese, grated

Directions:

1. Peel back the corn husks, remove silk strings and rinse corn under cold water.

2. Wrap 2 pieces of bacon around each ear of corn, securing with toothpicks.

3. Dust each ear of corn with some chili powder and cracked black pepper.

4. Supply your smoker with wood pellets and follow the start-up procedure. Preheat the grill, with the lid closed, to 375° F.

5. Place the ears of corn directly on the Traeger and grill for approximately 20 minutes or until the bacon is cooked crisp. Grill: 375 °F

6. Take the corn off the Traeger. Carefully remove the toothpicks and season with a little more chili powder and a grating of parmesan cheese, if desired. Serve & enjoy!

Grilled Corn On The Cob With Parmesan And Garlic

Servings: 6

Cooking Time: 30 Minutes

Ingredients:

➢ 4 Tablespoon butter, melted

➢ 2 Clove garlic, minced

➢ salt and pepper

➢ 8 ears fresh corn

➢ 1/2 Cup shaved Parmesan

➢ 1 Tablespoon chopped parsley

Directions:

1. Supply your smoker with wood pellets and follow the start-up procedure. Preheat the grill, with the lid closed, to 450° F.

2. Place butter, garlic, salt and pepper in a medium bowl and mix well.

3. Peel back corn husks and remove the silk. Rub corn with half of the garlic butter mixture.

4. Close husks and place directly on the grill grate. Cook for 25 to 30 minutes, turning occasionally until corn is tender. Grill: 450 °F

5. Remove from grill, peel and discard husks. Place corn on serving tray, drizzle with remaining butter and top with Parmesan and parsley.

Grilled Ratatouille Salad

Servings: 4

Cooking Time: 25 Minutes

Ingredients:

- ➤ 1 Whole sweet potatoes
- ➤ 1 Whole red onion, diced
- ➤ 1 Whole zucchini
- ➤ 1 Whole Squash
- ➤ 1 Large Tomato, diced
- ➤ vegetable oil
- ➤ salt and pepper

Directions:

1. Supply your smoker with wood pellets and follow the start-up procedure. Preheat the grill, with the lid closed, to High heat.

2. Slice all vegetables to a ¼ inch thickness.

3. Lightly brush each vegetable with oil and season with Traeger's Veggie Shake or salt and pepper.

4. Place sweet potato, onion, zucchini, and squash on grill grate and grill for 20 minutes or until tender, turn halfway through.

5. Add tomato slices to the grill during the last 5 minutes of cooking time.

6. For presentation, alternate vegetables while layering them vertically. Enjoy!

Cast Iron Potatoes

Servings: 4

Cooking Time: 60 Minutes

Ingredients:

➢ 4 Tablespoon butter, cut into cubes

➢ 2 1/2 Pound potatoes, peeled and cut into 1/8 inch slices

➢ 1/2 Large sweet onion, thinly sliced

➢ salt

➢ black pepper

➢ 1 1/2 Cup grated mild cheddar or jack cheese

➢ 2 Cup milk

➢ paprika

Directions:

1. Butter the inside of a cast iron skillet and layer half the potato slices on the bottom. Top with half the onions. Season with salt and pepper.

2. Sprinkle 1 cup of the cheese over the potatoes and onions and dot with half the butter. Layer the remaining potatoes and onions on top. Dot with remaining butter.

3. Pour the milk into the skillet. Cover the skillet tightly with aluminum foil.

4. Supply your smoker with wood pellets and follow the start-up procedure. Preheat the grill, with the lid closed, to 350° F.

5. Bake for 1 hour, or until the potatoes are very tender. Grill: 350 °F

6. Remove the foil and top with the remaining 1/2 cup of cheese. Bake for 30 minutes more (uncovered) until the cheese is lightly browned. Dust the top with paprika and serve immediately.

Roasted Hasselback Potatoes By Doug Scheiding

Servings: 6

Cooking Time: 120 Minutes

Ingredients:

- ➢ 6 Large russet potatoes
- ➢ 1 Pound bacon
- ➢ 1/2 Cup butter
- ➢ salt
- ➢ black pepper
- ➢ 1 Cup cheddar cheese
- ➢ 3 Whole scallions

Directions:

1. To cut potatoes, place two wooden spoons on either side of the potato (this prevents your knife from going all the way through). Slice potato into thin chips leaving about 1/4" attached on the bottom.

2. Freeze bacon slices for about 30 minutes then cut into small pieces about the size of a stamp. Place these in the cracks between every other slice.

3. Place the potato in a large cast iron skillet. Top the potato with slices of hard butter (you can also place thin slivers of cold butter between the potato slices with the bacon if desired). Season with salt and pepper.

4. Supply your smoker with wood pellets and follow the start-up procedure. Preheat the grill, with the lid closed, to 350° F.

5. Place the cast iron directly on the grill grate and cook for two hours. Top potatoes with more butter and baste with melted butter every 30 minutes.

6. In the last 10 minutes of cooking, sprinkle with cheddar and return to grill to melt.

7. To finish, top with chives or scallions. Enjoy!

Roasted Asparagus

Servings: 4

Cooking Time: 30 Minutes

Ingredients:

➢ 1 Bunch asparagus

➢ 2 Tablespoon olive oil, plus more as needed

➢ Veggie Rub

Directions:

1. Coat asparagus with olive oil and Veggie Rub, stirring to coat all pieces.

2. Supply your smoker with wood pellets and follow the start-up procedure. Preheat the grill, with the lid closed, to 350° F.

3. Place asparagus directly on the grill grate for 15-20 minutes.

4. Remove from grill and enjoy!

Roasted Sheet Pan Vegetables

Servings: 4

Cooking Time: 25 Minutes

Ingredients:

➢ 1 Small head purple cauliflower, stemmed and cut into 2 inch florets

➢ 1 Small head yellow cauliflower, stemmed and cut into 2 inch florets

➢ 4 Cup butternut squash

➢ 2 Cup oyster or shiitake mushrooms, rinsed and sliced

➢ 3 Tablespoon olive oil

➢ 2 Teaspoon kosher salt

➢ freshly ground black pepper

➢ 1/4 Cup chopped flat-leaf parsley

Directions:

1. Supply your smoker with wood pellets and follow the start-up procedure. Preheat the grill, with the lid closed, to 450° F.

2. In a large mixing bowl, combine all of the vegetables. Drizzle olive oil over the top, along with kosher salt and a generous grinding of black pepper.

3. Using your hands, toss the vegetables until they are evenly coated.

4. Spread out onto 1 or 2 half sheet pans or baking sheets, ensuring there is a little space between the veggies. (If they are too crowded, the vegetables will steam instead of roast and you won't get that crispy texture.)

5. Place the sheet pans on the grill and cook for 15 minutes. Open and stir, then close the lid and continue to cook until the vegetables are brown around the edges, about 5 to 15 minutes longer. Grill: 450 °F

6. Toss with parsley and serve immediately. The vegetables are also delicious at room temperature. Enjoy!

Smoked Beet-pickled Eggs

Servings: 4

Cooking Time: 30 Minutes

Ingredients:

➢ 6 Eggs, hard boiled
➢ 1 Red Beets, scrubbed and trimmed
➢ 1 Cup apple cider vinegar
➢ 1 Cup Beet, juice
➢ 1/4 Onion, Sliced
➢ 1/3 Cup granulated sugar
➢ 3 Cardamom
➢ 1 star anise

Directions:

1. Supply your smoker with wood pellets and follow the start-up procedure. Preheat the grill, with the lid closed, to 275° F.

2. Place the peeled hard boiled eggs directly on the grill and smoke for 30 minutes. Grill: 275 ˚F

3. Put the smoked eggs in a quart size glass jar with the cooked/chopped beets in the bottom.

4. In a medium sauce pan, add the vinegar, beet juice, onion, sugar, cardamom and anise.

5. Bring to a boil and cook, uncovered, until sugar has dissolved and the onions are translucent (about 5 minutes).

6. Remove from the heat and let cool for a few minutes.

7. Pour the vinegar and onions mixture over the eggs and beets in the jar, covering the eggs completely.

8. Securely close with the jar lid. Refrigerate up to a month. Enjoy!

POULTRY RECIPES

Jalapeno Chicken Sliders

Servings: 8-10

Cooking Time: 180 Minutes

Ingredients:

- ➢ 3 Pounds Boneless Skinless Chicken Breasts
- ➢ 8-10 Slices Cheese Of Choice
- ➢ 1/2 Cup Chicken Broth
- ➢ Pickled Jalapeños
- ➢ 1 Tsp Smoked Infused Sweet Mesquite Jalapeno Sea Salt
- ➢ 1/2 Cup Salsa Verde
- ➢ 1 Package Slider Buns
- ➢ 3 Tablespoons Sweet Heat Rub

Directions:

1. Add the chicken breasts, chicken broth, and salsa verde to a disposable aluminum foil pan. Season everything generously with Sweet Heat and 1 tsp of Smoked Infused Sweet Mesquite Jalapeno Sea Salt Cover tightly with aluminum foil.

2. Supply your smoker with wood pellets and follow the start-up procedure. Preheat the grill, with the lid open, to 275° F. Place the aluminum foil pan on the grill and cook for 3-4 hours, or until the chicken is completely cooked (165°F internal temperature), tender, and falling apart. Remove from the grill and let cool slightly.

3. Shred the chicken with the meat claws and toss with the Sweet Heat rub. Then, build the sliders: top the slider buns with a scoop of the pulled chicken, a slice cheese, and a few slices of pickled jalapeños Serve immediately.

Bbq Breakfast Sausage

Servings: 4 - 6

Cooking Time: 35 Minutes

Ingredients:

- 1/4 Cup Bbq Sauce
- 1 Tbsp Brown Sugar
- 4 Oz Cheddar Cheese, Cut Into Sticks
- To Taste, Cracked Black Pepper
- 6 Eggs, Scrambled
- 4 Oz Ham, Diced
- 1 Package, Approx 1 Lb Shady Brook Farms Ground Turkey Sausage
- 10 Oz Turkey Bacon

Directions:

1. Supply your smoker with wood pellets and follow the start-up procedure. Preheat the grill, with the lid closed, to 375° F. If using a gas or charcoal grill, set it up for medium-high heat.

2. Lay out a piece of plastic wrap then make a bacon weave using your favorite turkey bacon. Top with the Shady Brooks Farms Turkey Sausage and spread out into an even layer with your fingers.

3. Spoon the scrambled eggs into the center of the sausage, then place half of the cheese sticks in the middle, followed by ham, then remaining cheese.

4. Gently lift up one end of the plastic wrap and begin rolling the "not so fatty." Once the roll is completed, remove the plastic wrap and secure the ends of the bacon together with toothpicks, if needed.

5. Set in a cast iron skillet, sprinkle with brown sugar, and season with cracked pepper. Transfer to the grill and cook for 30 minutes, until an internal temperature of 155°F.

6. Baste with BBQ sauce and cook for an additional 5 minutes until the sauce is set and the internal temperature increased to 165°F.

7. Remove from the grill and rest for 5 minutes before slicing and serving warm.

Grilled Honey Chicken Kabobs

Servings: 4

Cooking Time: 14 Minutes

Ingredients:

➤ 1 pound boneless skinless chicken breasts (cut into 1 inch pieces)

➤ 1/4 cup olive oil

➤ 1/3 cup soy sauce

➤ 1/4 cup honey

➤ 1 teaspoon minced garlic

➤ salt and pepper to taste

➤ 1 red bell pepper (cut into 1 inch pieces)

➤ 1 yellow bell pepper (cut into 1 inch pieces)

➤ 2 small zucchini (cut into 1 inch slices)

➤ 1 red onion (cut into 1 inch pieces)

➤ 1 tablespoon chopped parsley

Directions:

1. In a large bowl combine the olive oil, soy sauce, honey, garlic and salt and pepper, and whisk.

2. Add the chicken, bell peppers, zucchini and red onion to the bowl, tossing to thoroughly coat.

3. Cover and refrigerate for 1 to 8 hours.

4. Soak wooden skewers in cold water for at least 30 minutes. Supply your smoker with wood pellets and follow the start-up procedure. Preheat the grill, with the lid closed, to high heat.

5. Thread the chicken and vegetables onto the skewers.

6. Cook for 5-7 minutes on each side or until chicken is cooked through.

7. To serve, sprinkle with parsley. Enjoy!

Bacon Wrapped Turkey Legs

Servings: 8

Cooking Time: 180 Minutes

Ingredients:

➢ 1 Gallon water

➢ 1/4 Cup Rub

➢ 3 Cup Morton Tender Quick Home Meat Cure

➢ 1/2 Cup brown sugar

➢ 6 Whole black peppercorns

➢ 2 Whole bay leaves

➢ 8 (1-1/2 lb each) turkey legs

➢ 8 Slices bacon

Directions:

1. Plan ahead, these turkey legs brine overnight. In a large stockpot, combine one gallon of water, Traeger Rub, curing salt, brown sugar, peppercorns and bay leaves.

2. Bring to a boil over high heat to dissolve the salt and sugar granules. Take off of the heat and add in 1/2 gallon of water and ice. Make sure the brine is at least to room temperature, if not colder. (You may need to refrigerate the brine for an hour or so.)

3. Add the turkey legs making sure they are completely submerged in the brine.

4. After 24 hours, drain the turkey legs and discard the brine. Rinse the brine off the legs with cold water, then dry thoroughly with paper towels.

5. Supply your smoker with wood pellets and follow the start-up procedure. Preheat the grill, with the lid closed, to 250° F.

6. Lay the turkey legs directly on the grill grate.

7. After 2-1/2 hours, wrap a piece of bacon around each leg and finish cooking them for the last 30 to 40 minutes. Grill: 250 ℉

8. The total cooking time for the legs will be 3 hours, or until the internal temperature reaches 165°F on an instant-read meat thermometer. Serve and enjoy! Grill: 250 ℉ Probe: 165 ℉

Fig Glazed Chicken Stuffed Cornbread

Servings: 10   Cooking Time: 120 Minutes

Ingredients:

- Black Pepper
- 6 Tablespoons (For The Chicken) Butter, Unsalted
- 3 Chicken, Whole
- 2 1/5 Cups (Replace With Craisins For A Different Flavor) Dried Figs, Chopped
- 1 Egg
- 2 Tablespoon Extra-Virgin Olive Oil
- 1/2 Cup Heavy Cream
- 1/2 Cup Honey
- Kosher Salt
- 4 Tablespoon Lemon, Juice
- 1/2 Onion, Chopped
- Champion Chicken Seasoning
- 1 1/2 Teaspoon Finely Chopped Rosemary, Fresh
- 1 Pound Sweet Italian Sausage
- 3 Cups Water, Warm

Directions:

1. Mix figs, honey, lemon juice, and warm water. Cover with plastic wrap and let figs soften for 30 minutes. Strain the figs and reserve the liquid for glaze.

2. Heat olive oil over medium heat and sauté the onions with rosemary. Add the sausage. Cook until browned. Place into a large bowl, add the cornbread and figs. Season with Champion Chicken Seasoning. Stir. In a separate bowl, Stir together egg, heavy whipping cream, and chicken stock. Pour over the cornbread/fig mix and stir together. Set aside.

3. Rinse chickens and pat dry. Season liberally with Champion Chicken Seasoning, kosher salt and black pepper. Don't forget the cavity! Stuff cavities with Stuffing. Top each Chicken with 2 tablespoons butter.

4. Supply your smoker with wood pellets and follow the start-up procedure. Preheat the grill, with the lid closed, to 300° F. Place in a roasting tray and cook until internal temp reads 165°F.

5. While chickens cook, place the fig liquid, balsamic vinegar and butter over. Reduce to thicken and baste chickens with about 160°F or 10 minutes before finished. Rest for 10 minutes. Carve and serve!

Grilled Cheesy Chicken

Servings: 4

Cooking Time: 45 Minutes

Ingredients:

➢ 4 Aged Chedder Cheese, Sliced
➢ 32 Oz Chicken Broth
➢ 1 Tsp Extra-Virgin Olive Oil
➢ Sweet Heat Rub And Grill
➢ 4 Plump Chicken, Boneless/Skinless

Directions:

1. Supply your smoker with wood pellets and follow the start-up procedure. Preheat the grill, with the lid open, to 350° F.

2. Remove the chicken from the brine. Pat the breasts dry and lightly brush olive oil on both sides of the chicken. Take your knife and slice diagonally across the top of each breast. Sprinkle a lit amount of Sweet Heat Rub and Grill on each side.

3. Barbecue your chicken breasts for 30 minutes. Next, place a slice of cheddar cheese on top of each breast.

4. Heat for another 5-10 minutes or until the cheese has fully melted into the incisions you made earlier. Remove and serve for a tender chicken breast with a spicy kick and hot cheesy center. You'll receive too much credit for a recipe this easy.

Roasted Rosemary Orange Chicken

Servings: 4

Cooking Time: 45 Minutes

Ingredients:

- 1 (3-4 lb) chicken, backbone removed
- 1/4 Cup olive oil
- 2 oranges, juiced
- 1 orange, zested
- 2 Teaspoon Dijon mustard
- 3 Tablespoon chopped rosemary leaves
- 2 Teaspoon kosher salt

Directions:

1. Rinse the chicken and pat dry with paper towels.

2. For the Marinade: In a medium bowl, combine olive oil, juice from the oranges (about 1/4 cup of freshly squeezed juice), orange zest, Dijon mustard, rosemary and salt. Whisk to combine.

3. Place the chicken in a shallow baking dish large enough for chicken to be fully opened in one piece. Pour marinade over the chicken ensuring it is covered with the marinade.

4. Cover with plastic wrap and refrigerate for a minimum of 2 hours or up to overnight, turning once during the process.

5. Supply your smoker with wood pellets and follow the start-up procedure. Preheat the grill, with the lid closed, to 350° F.

6. Remove the chicken from the marinade and place on the Traeger, skin-side down.

7. Cook for 25 to 30 minutes until the skin is well-browned, then flip. Continue to grill chicken until the internal temperature of the breast reaches 165°F and the thigh reaches 175°F, about 5 to 15 minutes longer. Grill: 350 °F Probe: 165 °F

8. Let rest 10 minutes before carving. Enjoy!

Smoking Duck With Mandarin Glaze

Servings: 4

Cooking Time: 240 Minutes

Ingredients:

➢ 1 quart buttermilk

➢ 1 (5-pound) whole duck

➢ ¾ cup soy sauce

➢ ½ cup hoisin sauce

➢ ½ cup rice wine vinegar

➢ 2 tablespoons sesame oil

➢ 1 tablespoon freshly ground black pepper

➢ 1 tablespoon minced garlic

➢ Mandarin Glaze, for drizzling

Directions:

1. With a very sharp knife, remove as much fat from the duck as you can. Refrigerate or freeze the fat for later use.

2. Pour the buttermilk into a large container with a lid and submerge the whole duck in it. Cover and let brine in the refrigerator for 4 to 6 hours.

3. Supply your smoker with wood pellets and follow the start-up procedure. Preheat, with the lid closed, to 250°F.

4. Remove the duck from the buttermilk brine, then rinse it and pat dry with paper towels.

5. In a bowl, combine the soy sauce, hoisin sauce, vinegar, sesame oil, pepper, and garlic to form a paste. Reserve ¼ cup for basting.

6. Poke holes in the skin of the duck and rub the remaining paste all over and inside the cavity.

7. Place the duck on the grill breast-side down, close the lid, and smoke for about 4 hours, basting every hour with the reserved paste, until a meat thermometer inserted in the thickest part of the meat reads 165°F. Use aluminum foil to tent the duck in the last 30 minutes or so if it starts to brown too quickly.

8. To finish, drizzle with glaze.

The Grilled Chicken Challenge

Servings: 4

Cooking Time: 60 Minutes

Ingredients:

➢ 1 (4 lb) whole chicken

➢ Chicken Rub

Directions:

1. Supply your smoker with wood pellets and follow the start-up procedure. Preheat the grill, with the lid closed, to 375° F.

2. Rinse and pat dry the whole chicken (remove and discard giblets, if any). Lightly season the entire chicken, including the cavity with Traeger Chicken Rub (or similar rub of choice).

3. Place the chicken on the grill grate and cook for about 1 hour and 10 minutes. Remove chicken from grill when internal temperature of breast reaches 160°F . The temperature will continue to rise to 165°F as the chicken rests. Check temperature periodically throughout as cook times will vary based on the weight of the chicken. Grill: 375 °F Probe: 160 °F

4. Allow bird to rest until internal temperature of breast reaches 165°F , 15 to 20 minutes. Enjoy!

Roasted Stuffed Turkey Breast

Servings: 6

Cooking Time: 40 Minutes

Ingredients:

➢ 1 (4-5 lb) boneless turkey breast

➢ 5 Slices thick-cut bacon, chopped

➢ 3/4 Cup assorted mushrooms

➢ 1 Bunch scallions, chopped

➢ 1/8 Cup white wine

➢ 3 Tablespoon panko breadcrumbs

➢ salt

➢ black pepper

Directions:

1. Supply your smoker with wood pellets and follow the start-up procedure. Preheat the grill, with the lid closed, to 375° F.

2. Slice the turkey breast horizontally, making sure not to slice all the way through. Lay breast open flat.

3. Cook bacon in a skillet over medium heat until crispy. Remove bacon and set aside. Sauté mushrooms in the bacon grease until browned. Add scallions and cook for an additional two minutes. Add white wine and cook down until no wine remains. Stir in breadcrumbs and bacon, adding salt and pepper to taste.

4. Transfer filling to fridge to cool for 15 to 20 minutes. Once chilled, spread the filling onto the turkey breast, pressing lightly to make sure it adheres. Roll the turkey breast tightly and tie with butcher's twine at about 1 inch intervals. Tuck the ends of the turkey breast under and tie with twine lengthwise.

5. Season the outside of the turkey breast with salt and pepper. Place in grill for 40 minutes. Check the internal temperature, desired temperature is 165°F. Once the finished temperature is reached, remove turkey from the grill and let rest for 10 minutes. Slice and serve. Enjoy! Grill: 375 °F Probe: 165 °F

Bbq Game Day Chicken Wings And Thighs

Servings: 6

Cooking Time: 50 Minutes

Ingredients:

➢ 10 chicken thighs

➢ 30 chicken wings

➢ 1/2 Cup olive oil

➢ 1/2 Cup Chicken Rub

Directions:

1. Place thighs and wings in a large bowl. Add the olive oil and Traeger Chicken Rub and mix well. Cover bowl and refrigerate for 3 to 8 hours.

2. Supply your smoker with wood pellets and follow the start-up procedure. Preheat the grill, with the lid closed, to 375° F.

3. Place chicken directly on the grill grate and cook for 45 minutes. Check the internal temperature of the chicken, it is considered done at 165°F, however, a finished temperature of 175 to 180°F results in a better texture in dark meat. Grill: 375 °F Probe: 165 °F

4. Once the finished temperature is reached, remove chicken from the grill and let rest for 5 to 10 minutes before serving. Enjoy!

Traeger Bbq Half Chickens

Servings: 2

Cooking Time: 60 Minutes

Ingredients:

➤ 1 (3 to 3-1/2 lb) fresh young chicken

➤ Leinenkugel's Summer Shandy Rub

➤ Apricot BBQ Sauce

Directions:

1. Place the chicken breast side down, on a cutting board with the neck pointing away from you. Cut along one side of the backbone, staying as close to the bone as possible, from the neck to the tail. Repeat on the other side of the backbone then remove it.

2. Open the chicken and slice through the white cartilage at the tip of the breastbone to pop it open. Cut down either side of the breast bone then use your fingers to pull it out. Flip the chicken over so it is skin side up and cut down the center splitting the chicken in half. Tuck the wings back on each chicken half.

3. Season on both sides with Traeger Leinenkugel's Summer Shandy Rub.

4. Supply your smoker with wood pellets and follow the start-up procedure. Preheat the grill, with the lid closed, to 375° F.

5. Place chicken directly on the grill grate skin side up and cook until the internal temperature reaches 160°F, about 60-90 minutes. Grill: 375 °F Probe: 160 °F

6. Brush the BBQ sauce all over the chicken skin and cook for an additional 10 minutes. Remove from grill and let rest 5 minutes before serving. Enjoy! Grill: 375 °F

Apple Bacon Lattice Turkey

Servings: 7

Cooking Time: 180 Minutes

Ingredients:

- ➢ 2 Apples
- ➢ Bacon
- ➢ 2 Celery, Stick
- ➢ (Parsley, Rosemary, Thyme) Herb Mix
- ➢ 1 Onion, Sliced
- ➢ Pepper
- ➢ Grills Champion Chicken Seasoning
- ➢ 1 Brined Turkey

Directions:

1. Supply your smoker with wood pellets and follow the start-up procedure. Preheat the grill, with the lid closed, to 300° F.

2. Be sure all the innards and giblets of the turkey have been removed.

3. Wash the external and internal parts of the turkey and pat the surface dry with a paper towel.

4. Slice fruit and veggies into large chunks and stuff inside turkey.

5. Liberally season the whole Turkey with Champion Chicken Seasoning.

6. Prep bacon into lattice design on a flexible cutting board. Flip onto top of turkey, covering the breasts.

7. Season with more Champion Chicken and black pepper

8. Season with more Champion Chicken and black pepper

9. Let the turkey rest for 30 minutes.

APPETIZERS AND SNACKS

Citrus-infused Marinated Olives

Servings: 6

Cooking Time: 30 Minutes

Ingredients:

- 1½ cups mixed brined olives, with pits
- ½ cup extra virgin olive oil
- 1 tbsp freshly squeezed lemon juice
- 1 garlic clove, peeled and thinly sliced
- 1 tsp smoked Spanish paprika
- 2 sprigs of fresh rosemary
- 2 sprigs of fresh thyme
- 2 bay leaves, fresh or dried
- 1 small dried red chili pepper, deseeded and flesh crumbled, or ¼ tsp crushed red pepper flakes
- 3 strips of orange zest
- 3 strips of lemon zest

Directions:

1. Supply your smoker with wood pellets and follow the start-up procedure. Preheat the grill, with the lid closed, to 180° F.

2. Drain the olives, reserving 1 tablespoon of brine. Spread the olives in a single layer in an aluminum foil roasting pan. Place the pan on the grate and cook the olives for 30 minutes, stirring the olives or shaking the pan once or twice.

3. In a small saucepan on the stovetop over low heat, warm the olive oil. Whisk in the lemon juice and the reserved 1 tablespoon of brine. Stir in the garlic and paprika. Add the rosemary, thyme, bay leaves, chili pepper, and orange and lemon zests. Warm over low heat for 10 minutes. Remove the saucepan from the heat.

4. Transfer the olives and olive oil mixture to a pint jar. Tuck the aromatics around the sides of the jar. Let cool and then cover and refrigerate for up to 5 days. Let the olives come to room temperature before serving.

Roasted Red Pepper Dip

Servings: 8   Cooking Time: 45 Minutes

Ingredients:

- 4 red bell peppers, halved, destemmed, and deseeded
- 1 cup English walnuts, divided
- 1 small white onion, peeled and coarsely chopped
- 2 garlic cloves, peeled and smashed with a chef's knife
- ¼ cup extra virgin olive oil, plus more
- 1 tbsp balsamic vinegar or balsamic glaze
- 1 tsp honey (eliminate if using balsamic glaze)
- 1 tsp coarse salt, plus more
- 1 tsp ground cumin
- 1 tsp smoked paprika
- ½ to 1 tsp Aleppo red pepper flakes, plus more
- ¼ cup fresh white breadcrumbs (optional)
- distilled water (optional)
- assorted crudités or wedges of pita bread

Directions:

1. Supply your smoker with wood pellets and follow the start-up procedure. Preheat the grill, with the lid closed, to 400° F.

2. Place the peppers skin side down on the grate and grill until the skins blister and the flesh softens, about 30 minutes. Transfer the peppers to a bowl and cover with plastic wrap. Let cool to room temperature. Remove the skins with a paring knife or your fingers. Coarsely chop or tear the peppers.

3. Place ¾ cup of walnuts in an aluminum foil roasting pan. Place the pan on the grate and toast for 10 to 15 minutes, stirring twice. Remove the pan from the grill and let the walnuts cool.

4. Place the peppers, onion, garlic, and walnuts in a food processor fitted with the chopping blade. Pulse several times. Add the olive oil, balsamic vinegar, honey, salt, cumin, paprika, and red pepper flakes. Process until the mixture is fairly smooth. Taste for seasoning, adding more salt or red pepper flakes (if desired). (If the mixture is too loose, add breadcrumbs until the texture is to your liking. If it's too thick, add olive oil or water 1 tablespoon at a time.)

5. Transfer the dip to a serving bowl. Use the back of a spoon to make a shallow depression in the center. Top with the remaining ¼ cup of walnuts and drizzle olive oil in the depression. Serve with crudités or pita bread.

Pigs In A Blanket

Servings: 4-6

Cooking Time: 15 Minutes

Ingredients:

➢ 2 Tablespoon Poppy Seeds

➢ 1 Tablespoon Dried Minced Onion

➢ 2 Teaspoon garlic, minced

➢ 2 Tablespoon Sesame Seeds

➢ 1 Teaspoon salt

➢ 8 Ounce Original Crescent Dough

➢ 1/4 Cup Dijon mustard

➢ 1 Large egg, beaten

Directions:

1. When ready to cook, start your smoker at 350 degrees F, and preheat with lid closed, 10 to 15 minutes.

2. Mix together poppy seeds, dried minced onion, dried minced garlic, salt and sesame seeds. Set aside.

3. Cut each triangle of crescent roll dough into thirds lengthwise, making 3 small strips from each roll.

4. Brush the dough strips lightly with Dijon mustard. Put the mini hot dogs on 1 end of the dough and roll up.

5. Arrange them, seam side down, on a greased baking pan. Brush with egg wash and sprinkle with seasoning mixture.

6. Bake in smoker until golden brown, about 12 to 15 minutes.

7. Serve with mustard or dipping sauce of your choice. Enjoy!

Grilled Guacamole

Servings: 6

Cooking Time: 30 Minutes

Ingredients:

- ➤ 3 large avocados, halved and pitted
- ➤ 1 lime, halved
- ➤ ½ jalapeño, deseeded and deveined
- ➤ ½ small white or red onion, peeled
- ➤ 2 garlic cloves, peeled and skewered on a toothpick
- ➤ 1 tsp coarse salt, plus more
- ➤ 1½ tbsp reduced-fat mayo
- ➤ 2 tbsp chopped fresh cilantro
- ➤ 2 tbsp crumbled queso fresco (optional)
- ➤ tortilla chips

Directions:

1. Supply your smoker with wood pellets and follow the start-up procedure. Preheat the grill, with the lid closed, to 225° F.

2. Place the avocados, lime, jalapeño, and onion cut sides down on the grate. Use the toothpicks to balance the garlic cloves between the bars. Smoke for 30 minutes. (You want the vegetables to retain most of their rawness.)

3. Transfer everything to a cutting board. Remove the garlic cloves from the toothpick and roughly chop. Sprinkle with the salt and continue to mince the garlic until it begins to form a paste. Scrape the garlic and salt into a large bowl.

4. Scoop the avocado flesh from the peels into the bowl. Squeeze the juice of ½ lime over the avocado. Mash the avocados but leave them somewhat chunky. Finely dice the jalapeño. Dice 2 tablespoons of onion. (Reserve the remaining onion for another use.) Add the jalapeño, onion, mayo, and cilantro to the bowl. Stir gently to combine. Taste for seasoning, adding more salt, lime juice, and jalapeño as desired.

5. Transfer the guacamole to a serving bowl. Top with the queso fresco (if using). Serve with tortilla chips.

Cold-smoked Cheese

Servings: 6   Cooking Time: 180 Minutes

Ingredients:

- 2lb (1kg) well-chilled hard or semi-hard cheese, such as:
- Edam
- Gouda
- Cheddar
- Monterey Jack
- pepper Jack
- goat cheese
- fresh mozzarella
- Muenster
- aged Parmigiano-Reggiano
- Gruyère
- blue cheese

Directions:

1. Unwrap the cheese and remove any protective wax or coating. Cut into 4-ounce (110g) portions to increase the surface area.

2. If possible, move your smoker to a shady area. Place 1 resealable plastic bag filled with ice on top of the drip pan. This is especially important on a warm day because you want to keep the interior temperature of the grill between 70 and 90°F (21 and 32°C) or below.

3. Place a grill mat on one side of the grate. Place the cheese on the mat and allow space between each piece.

4. Fill your smoking tube or pellet maze (see Cast Iron Skillets and Grill Pans) with pellets or sawdust and light according to the manufacturer's instructions. Place the smoking tube on the grate near—but not on—the grill mat. When the tube is smoking consistently, close the grill lid.

5. Smoke the cheese for 1 to 3 hours, replacing the pellets or sawdust and ice if necessary. Monitor the temperature and make sure the cheese isn't beginning to melt. Carefully lift the mat with the cheese to a rimmed baking sheet and let the cheese cool completely before handling.

6. Package the smoked cheese in cheese storage paper or bags or vacuum-seal the cheese, labeling each. (While you can wrap the cheese tightly in plastic wrap, the cheese will spoil faster.) Let the cheese rest for at least 2 to 3 days before eating. It will be even better after 2 weeks.

Bacon Pork Pinwheels (kansas Lollipops)

Servings: 4-6

Cooking Time: 20 Minutes

Ingredients:

➢ 1 Whole Pork Loin, boneless

➢ To Taste salt and pepper

➢ To Taste Greek Seasoning

➢ 4 Slices bacon

➢ To Taste The Ultimate BBQ Sauce

Directions:

1. When ready to cook, start the smoker and set temperature to 500F. Preheat, lid closed, for 10 to 15 minutes.

2. Trim pork loin of any unwanted silver skin or fat. Using a sharp knife, cut pork loin length wise, into 4 long strips.

3. Lay pork flat, then season with salt, pepper and Cavender's Greek Seasoning.

4. Flip the pork strips over and layer bacon on unseasoned side. Begin tightly rolling the pork strips, with bacon being rolled up on the inside.

5. Secure a skewer all the way through each pork roll to secure it in place. Set the pork rolls down on grill and cook for 15 minutes.

6. Brush BBQ Sauce over the pork. Turn each skewer over, then coat the other side. Let pork cook for another 5-10 minutes, depending on thickness of your pork. Enjoy!

Chicken Wings With Teriyaki Glaze

Servings: 4   Cooking Time: 50 Minutes

Ingredients:

- 16 large chicken wings, about 3lb (1.4kg) total
- 1 to 1½ tbsp toasted sesame oil
- for the glaze
- ½ cup light soy sauce or tamari
- ¼ cup sake or sugar-free dark-colored soda
- ¼ cup light brown sugar or low-carb substitute
- 2 tbsp mirin or 1 tbsp honey

- 1 garlic clove, peeled, minced or grated
- 2 tsp minced fresh ginger
- 1 tsp cornstarch mixed with 1 tbsp distilled water (optional)
- for serving
- 1 tbsp toasted sesame seeds
- 2 scallions, trimmed, white and green parts sliced sharply diagonally

Directions:

1. Supply your smoker with wood pellets and follow the start-up procedure. Preheat the grill, with the lid closed, to 350° F.

2. Place the chicken wings in a large bowl, add the sesame oil, and turn the wings to coat thoroughly.

3. Place the wings on the grate at an angle to the bars. Grill for 20 minutes and then turn. Continue to cook until the wings are nicely browned and the meat is no longer pink at the bone, about 20 minutes more.

4. To make the glaze, in a saucepan on the stovetop over medium-high heat, combine the ingredients and bring the mixture to a boil. Reduce the glaze by 1⁄3, about 6 to 8 minutes. If you prefer your glaze to be glossy and thick, add the cornstarch and water mixture to the glaze and cook until it coats the back of a spoon, about 1 to 2 minutes more.

5. Transfer the wings to an aluminum foil roasting pan. Pour the glaze over them, turning to coat thoroughly. Place the pan on the grate and cook the wings until the glaze sets, about 5 to 10 minutes.

6. Transfer the wings to a platter. Scatter the sesame seeds and scallions over the top. Serve with plenty of napkins.

Bacon-wrapped Jalapeño Poppers

Servings: 12

Cooking Time: 30 Minutes

Ingredients:

- ➤ 8 ounces cream cheese, softened
- ➤ ½ cup shredded Cheddar cheese
- ➤ ¼ cup chopped scallions
- ➤ 1 teaspoon chipotle chile powder or regular chili powder
- ➤ 1 teaspoon garlic powder
- ➤ 1 teaspoon salt
- ➤ 18 large jalapeño peppers, stemmed, seeded, and halved lengthwise
- ➤ 1 pound bacon (precooked works well)

Directions:

1. Supply your smoker with wood pellets and follow the start-up procedure. Preheat, with the lid closed, to 350°F. Line a baking sheet with aluminum foil.

2. In a small bowl, combine the cream cheese, Cheddar cheese, scallions, chipotle powder, garlic powder, and salt.

3. Stuff the jalapeño halves with the cheese mixture.

4. Cut the bacon into pieces big enough to wrap around the stuffed pepper halves.

5. Wrap the bacon around the peppers and place on the prepared baking sheet.

6. Put the baking sheet on the grill grate, close the lid, and smoke the peppers for 30 minutes, or until the cheese is melted and the bacon is cooked through and crisp.

7. Let the jalapeño poppers cool for 3 to 5 minutes. Serve warm.

Smoked Cashews

Servings: 6

Cooking Time: 60 Minutes

Ingredients:

➢ 1 pound roasted, salted cashews

Directions:

1. Supply your smoker with wood pellets and follow the start-up procedure. Preheat the grill, with the lid closed, to 120°F.

2. Pour the cashews onto a rimmed baking sheet and smoke for 1 hour, stirring once about halfway through the smoking time.

3. Remove the cashews from the grill, let cool, and store in an airtight container for as long as you can resist.

Deviled Eggs With Smoked Paprika

Servings: 6

Cooking Time: 30 Minutes

Ingredients:

- 6 large eggs
- 3 tbsp reduced-fat mayo, plus more
- 1 tsp Dijon or yellow mustard
- ½ tsp Spanish smoked paprika or regular paprika, plus more
- dash of hot sauce
- coarse salt
- freshly ground black pepper
- for garnishing
- small sprigs of fresh parsley, dill, tarragon, or cilantro
- chopped chives
- minced scallions
- Mustard Caviar
- sliced green or black olives
- celery leaves
- sliced radishes
- diced bell peppers
- sliced cherry tomatoes
- fresh or pickled jalapeños
- sliced or diced pickles
- slivers of sun-dried tomatoes
- bacon crumbles
- smoked salmon
- Hawaiian black salt
- Caviar

Directions:

1. Supply your smoker with wood pellets and follow the start-up procedure. Preheat the grill, with the lid closed, to 180° F.

2. On the stovetop over medium-high heat, bring a saucepan of water to a boil. (Make sure there's enough water in the saucepan to cover the eggs by 1 inch [5cm].) Use a slotted spoon to gently lower the eggs into the water. Lower the heat to maintain a simmer. Set a timer for 13 minutes.

3. Prepare an ice bath by combining ice and cold water in a large bowl. Carefully transfer the eggs to the ice bath when the timer goes off.

4. When the eggs are cool enough to handle, gently tap them all over to crack the shell. Carefully peel the eggs. Rinse under cold running water to remove any clinging bits of shell, but don't dry the eggs. (A damp surface will help the smoke adhere to the egg whites.)

5. Place the eggs on the grate and smoke until the eggs take on a light brown patina from the smoke, about 25 minutes. Transfer the eggs to a cutting board, handling them as little as possible.

6. Slice each egg in half lengthwise with a sharp knife. Wipe any yolk off the blade before slicing the next egg. Gently remove the yolks and place them in a food processor. Pulse to break up the yolks. Add the mayo, mustard, paprika, and hot sauce. Season with salt and pepper to taste. Pulse until the filling is

smooth. Add additional mayo 1 teaspoon at a time if the mixture is a little dry. (It shouldn't be too loose either.)

7. Spoon the filling into each egg half or pipe it in using a small resealable plastic bag. You can also use a pastry bag fitted with a fluted tip.

8. Place the eggs on a platter and lightly dust with paprika. Accompany with one or more of the suggested garnishes.

Sriracha & Maple Cashews

Servings: 10

Cooking Time: 60 Minutes

Ingredients:

➢ 2 tbsp unsalted butter

➢ 3 tbsp pure maple syrup

➢ 1 tbsp sriracha

➢ 1 tsp coarse salt (use only if nuts are unsalted)

➢ 2½ cups unsalted cashews

Directions:

1. Supply your smoker with wood pellets and follow the start-up procedure. Preheat the grill, with the lid closed, to 250° F.

2. In a small saucepan on the stovetop over low heat, melt the butter. Add the maple syrup, sriracha, and salt (if using). Stir until combined. Add the nuts and stir gently to coat thoroughly.

3. Spread the nuts in a single layer in an aluminum foil roasting pan coated with cooking spray. Place the pan on the grate and smoke the nuts until they're lightly toasted, about 1 hour, stirring once or twice.

4. Remove the pan from the grill and let the nuts cool for 15 minutes. They'll be sticky at first but will crisp up. Break them up with your fingers and store at room temperature in an airtight container, such as a lidded glass jar.

Jalapeño Poppers With Chipotle Sour Cream

Servings: 8   Cooking Time: 45 Minutes

Ingredients:

- 3 strips of thin-sliced bacon
- 12 large jalapeños, red, green, or a mix
- 8oz (225g) light cream cheese, at room temperature
- 1 cup shredded pepper Jack, Monterey Jack, or Cheddar cheese
- 1 tsp chili powder
- ½ tsp garlic salt
- smoked paprika

- for the sour cream
- 1¼ cups light sour cream
- juice of ½ lime
- ½ to 1 canned chipotle peppers in adobo sauce, finely minced, plus 1 tsp of sauce, plus more
- 1 tbsp minced fresh cilantro leaves
- ½ tsp coarse salt, plus more

Directions:

1. Supply your smoker with wood pellets and follow the start-up procedure. Preheat the grill, with the lid closed, to 375° F.

2. Line a rimmed sheet pan with aluminum foil and place a wire rack on top. Place the bacon in a single layer on the wire rack. Place the pan on the grate and grill until the bacon is crisp and golden brown, about 20 minutes. Transfer the bacon to paper towels to cool and then crumble. Set aside.

3. In a small bowl, make the chipotle sour cream by whisking together the ingredients. Add more salt, chipotle peppers, or adobe sauce to taste. Cover and refrigerate.

4. Slice the jalapeños lengthwise through their stems. Scrape out the veins and seeds with the edge of a small metal spoon.

5. In a small bowl, beat together the cream cheese, shredded cheese, chili powder, and garlic salt. Stir in the crumbled bacon. Mound the cream cheese mixture in the jalapeño halves. Line another rimmed sheet pan with aluminum foil and place a wire rack on top. Place the jalapeños filled side up in a single layer on the wire rack.

6. Place the sheet pan on the grate and roast the jalapeños until the filling has melted and the peppers have softened, about 20 to 25 minutes. (They should no longer look bright in color.) Remove the pan from the grill and let the peppers rest for 5 minutes.

7. Transfer the poppers to a platter and lightly dust with paprika. Serve with the chipotle sour cream.

Pulled Pork Loaded Nachos

Servings: 4   Cooking Time: 10 Minutes

Ingredients:

- 2 cups leftover smoked pulled pork
- 1 small sweet onion, diced
- 1 medium tomato, diced
- 1 jalapeño pepper, seeded and diced
- 1 garlic clove, minced
- 1 teaspoon salt
- 1 teaspoon freshly ground black pepper
- 1 bag tortilla chips

- 1 cup shredded Cheddar cheese
- ½ cup The Ultimate BBQ Sauce, divided
- ½ cup shredded jalapeño Monterey Jack cheese
- Juice of ½ lime
- 1 avocado, halved, pitted, and sliced
- 2 tablespoons sour cream
- 1 tablespoon chopped fresh cilantro

Directions:

1. Supply your smoker with wood pellets and follow the start-up procedure. Preheat, with the lid closed, to 375°F.

2. Heat the pulled pork in the microwave.

3. In a medium bowl, combine the onion, tomato, jalapeño, garlic, salt, and pepper, and set aside.

4. Arrange half of the tortilla chips in a large cast iron skillet. Spread half of the warmed pork on top and cover with the Cheddar cheese. Top with half of the onion-jalapeño mixture, then drizzle with ¼ cup of barbecue sauce.

5. Layer on the remaining tortilla chips, then the remaining pork and the Monterey Jack cheese. Top with the remaining onion-jalapeño mixture and drizzle with the remaining ¼ cup of barbecue sauce.

6. Place the skillet on the grill, close the lid, and smoke for about 10 minutes, or until the cheese is melted and bubbly. (Watch to make sure your chips don't burn!)

7. Squeeze the lime juice over the nachos, top with the avocado slices and sour cream, and garnish with the cilantro before serving hot.

COCKTAILS RECIPES

Smoked Pomegranate Lemonade Cocktail

Servings: 2

Cooking Time: 45 Minutes

Ingredients:

- ➢ 32 Ounce POM Juice
- ➢ 2 Cup pomegranate seeds
- ➢ 3 Ounce vodka
- ➢ 8 Ounce lemonade
- ➢ lemon wheel, for garnish
- ➢ fresh mint, for garnish

Directions:

1. Supply your smoker with wood pellets and follow the start-up procedure. Preheat the grill, with the lid closed, to 225° F.

2. For the Smoked Pomegranate Ice Cubes: Pour one small container of POM juice and 1 cup of pomegranate seeds into a shallow sheet pan. Smoke on the Traeger for 45 minutes. Pull off grill and let sit until cooled. Grill: 180 °F

3. Pour smoked POM juice into ice molds of your choice and put into freezer.

4. When ready to serve, place the frozen pomegranate cubes into a mason jar. Pour vodka and lemonade over the ice cubes.

5. Garnish with a lemon wheel and fresh mint. Enjoy!

In Traeger Fashion Cocktail

Servings: 2

Cooking Time: 20 Minutes

Ingredients:

➢ 2 Whole orange peel

➢ 2 Whole lemon peel

➢ 3 Ounce bourbon

➢ 1 Ounce Smoked Simple Syrup

➢ 6 Dash Bitters Lab Charred Cedar & Currant Bitters

Directions:

1. Supply your smoker with wood pellets and follow the start-up procedure. Preheat the grill, with the lid closed, to 350° F.

2. Place the lemon and orange peel directly on the grill grate and cook 20 to 25 minutes or until lightly browned. Grill: 350 °F

3. Add bourbon, Traeger Smoked Simple Syrup and bitters to a mixing glass and stir over ice. Stir until glass is chilled and contents are well diluted.

4. Strain into a new glass over fresh ice and garnish with grilled lemon and orange peel. Enjoy!

Smoked Texas Ranch Water

Servings: 4

Cooking Time: 60 Minutes

Ingredients:

- ➢ 3 Whole limes
- ➢ 1 Tablespoon Blackened Saskatchewan Rub
- ➢ 12 Ounce blanco tequila
- ➢ 24 Ounce Topo Chico or other sparkling mineral water
- ➢ 8 Slices jalapeño, optional

Directions:

1. Supply your smoker with wood pellets and follow the start-up procedure. Preheat the grill, with the lid closed, to 225° F.

2. Cut two of the limes in half and sprinkle with Traeger Blackened Saskatchewan Rub. Place the four lime halves on the edge of the grill grate and smoke for 1 hour. Remove from grill and set aside to cool. Grill: 225 °F

3. Pour some of the rub onto a small plate. Cut the third lime into 1/4 wedges and use the lime to rub the rim of 4 cocktail glasses, turn the glasses upside down, and into the rub to salt the rim.

4. Place several ice cubes into your rimmed glasses and pour 3 ounces tequila, 6 ounces Topo Chico, squeeze the juice of one smoked lime (discard after squeezing), and add one fresh lime wedge to each. If using the jalapeño, add one or two slices to each glass (muddle if desired).

5. Stir to combine and enjoy!

Sunset Margarita

Servings: 2

Cooking Time: 55 Minutes

Ingredients:

➢ 4 oranges

➢ 2 Cup plus 1 teaspoon agave

➢ 1/2 Cup water

➢ 1 Ounce burnt orange agave

➢ 3 Ounce reposado tequila

➢ 1 1/2 Ounce fresh squeezed lime juice

➢ Jacobsen Salt Co. Cherrywood Smoked Salt

Directions:

1. Supply your smoker with wood pellets and follow the start-up procedure. Preheat the grill, with the lid closed, to 350° F.

2. For the Burnt Orange Agave Syrup: Cut one orange in half and brush cut side with agave. Place cut side down directly on the grill grate and grill for 15 minutes or until grill marks develop. Grill: 350 °F

3. While the orange halves are grilling, slice the other orange and brush both sides of the slices with agave. Place slices directly on the grill grate next to the halves and cook for 15 minutes or until grill marks develop. Grill: 350 °F

4. Remove orange halves from grill grate and let cool. After they have cooled, juice halves and strain. Set aside.

5. Combine 1/4 cup water and agave in a shallow dish and mix well. Remove orange slices from the grill and place in the agave mixture, reserving a few for garnish.

6. Reduce the grill temperature to 180 degrees F and place the shallow dish with agave and oranges directly on the grill grate. Smoke for 40 minutes. Remove from heat and strain. Set aside. Grill: 180 °F

7. To Mix Drink: Rim glass with Jacobsen Smoked Salt. Combine tequila, fresh lime juice, grilled orange juice and burnt orange agave syrup in a glass. Add ice and shake well.

8. Strain into a rimmed glass over clean ice. Garnish with a grilled orange slice. Enjoy!

Strawberry Mule Cocktail

Servings: 2

Cooking Time: 15 Minutes

Ingredients:

➢ 8 grilled strawberries, plus more for serving

➢ 3 Ounce vodka

➢ 1 Ounce Smoked Simple Syrup

➢ 1 Ounce lemon juice

➢ 6 Ounce ginger beer

➢ fresh mint leaves

Directions:

1. Supply your smoker with wood pellets and follow the start-up procedure. Preheat the grill, with the lid closed, to 400° F.

2. Place strawberries directly on the grill grate and cook 15 minutes or until grill marks appear. Grill: 400 ˚F

3. For the cocktail: Add vodka, grilled strawberries, Traeger Smoked Simple Syrup and lemon juice to a shaker. Shake vigorously.

4. Double strain into a fresh glass or copper mug with crushed ice.

5. Top with ginger beer and garnish with extra grilled strawberries and fresh mint. Enjoy!

Batter Up Cocktail

Servings: 2

Cooking Time: 60 Minutes

Ingredients:

➢ 2 whole nutmeg

➢ 4 Ounce Michter's Bourbon

➢ 3 Teaspoon pumpkin puree

➢ 1 Ounce Smoked Simple Syrup

➢ 2 Large egg

Directions:

1. Supply your smoker with wood pellets and follow the start-up procedure. Preheat the grill, with the lid closed, to 180° F.

2. Place whole nutmeg on a sheet tray and place in the grill. Smoke 1 hour. Remove from grill and let cool. Grill: 180 °F

3. Add everything to a shaker and shake without ice. Add ice, then shake and strain into a chilled highball glass.

4. Garnish with grated, smoked nutmeg. Enjoy!

Smoked Ice Mojito Slurpee

Servings: 2

Cooking Time: 30 Minutes

Ingredients:

- ➢ water
- ➢ 1 Cup white rum
- ➢ 1/2 Cup lime juice
- ➢ 1/4 Cup Smoked Simple Syrup
- ➢ 12 Whole fresh mint leaves
- ➢ 4 Sprig mint
- ➢ 4 Whole lime wedge, for garnish

Directions:

1. Supply your smoker with wood pellets and follow the start-up procedure. Preheat the grill, with the lid closed, to 180° F.
2. For optimal flavor, use Super Smoke if available. Grill: 180 °F
3. Remove water from grill and pour smoked water into ice cube trays. Place in freezer until frozen.
4. Add rum, lime juice, Traeger Smoked Simple Syrup, mint and smoked ice to a blender.
5. Blend until a slushy consistency and pour into glasses.
6. Garnish with a mint sprig and lime wedge. Enjoy!

Zombie Cocktail Recipe

Servings: 2

Cooking Time: 45 Minutes

Ingredients:

➢ fresh squeezed orange juice

➢ pineapple juice

➢ 2 Ounce light rum

➢ 2 Ounce dark rum

➢ 2 Ounce lime juice

➢ 1 Ounce Smoked Simple Syrup

➢ 6 Ounce smoked orange and pineapple juice

➢ 2 grilled orange peel, for garnish

➢ 2 grilled pineapple chunks, for garnish

Directions:

1. Supply your smoker with wood pellets and follow the start-up procedure. Preheat the grill, with the lid closed, to 180° F.

2. Smoked Orange and Pineapple Juice: Pour equal parts fresh squeezed orange juice and pineapple juice into a shallow sheet pan and smoke for 45 minutes. Remove and let cool. Measure out 3 ounces of juice and reserve any remaining juice in the refrigerator for future use. Grill: 180 °F

3. Add dark and light rums, 3 ounces smoked orange and pineapple juice, lime juice and Traeger Smoked Simple Syrup to a mixing glass.

4. Add ice, shake and strain over clean ice into a Tiki glass.

5. Garnish with a grilled orange peel and grilled pineapple. Enjoy!

Grilled Rabbit Tail Cocktail

Servings: 2

Cooking Time: 25 Minutes

Ingredients:

- ➢ 1 1/2 Ounce lemon juice
- ➢ 4 Ounce Apple Brandy
- ➢ 1 Ounce orange juice
- ➢ 1 Ounce Smoked Simple Syrup

Directions:

1. Supply your smoker with wood pellets and follow the start-up procedure. Preheat the grill, with the lid closed, to 350° F.

2. Place lemon halves directly on the grill grate and cook for 20-25 minutes or until grill marks appear. Remove from grill and let cool. Once cool enough to handle, juice the lemons then chill and reserve the juice. Grill: 350 °F

3. Using the proportions listed above and considering the size and consumption rate of your tailgate crew or party, mix all the above ingredients in a large thermos and top with a bit of ice.

4. Using 6-8 oz glasses or cups, guests can serve themselves from the thermos and garnish each drink with a grilled apple slice. Enjoy!

Smoked Barnburner Cocktail

Servings: 2

Cooking Time: 45 Minutes

Ingredients:

➢ 16 Ounce fresh raspberries

➢ 1/2 Cup Smoked Simple Syrup

➢ 1 1/2 Ounce smoked raspberry syrup

➢ 3 Ounce reposado tequila

➢ 1 Ounce lime juice

➢ 1 Ounce lemon juice

➢ 2 grilled lime wheel, for garnish

Directions:

1. Supply your smoker with wood pellets and follow the start-up procedure. Preheat the grill, with the lid closed, to 180° F.

2. For Smoked Raspberry Syrup: Place fresh raspberries on a grill mat and smoke for 30 minutes. After the raspberries have been smoked, reserve a few for garnish and place the remainder into a shallow sheet pan with Traeger Smoked Simple Syrup. Grill: 180 ˚F

3. Place sheet pan on the grill grate and smoke for 45 minutes. Remove from grill and let cool. Strain through a fine mesh sieve discarding solids. Transfer the syrup to the refrigerator until ready to use. Makes about 1/2 cup of smoked raspberry syrup. Grill: 180 ˚F

4. For cocktail: Add 3/4 ounce smoked raspberry syrup, tequila, lime juice and lemon juice with ice into a mixing glass. Shake and pour over clean ice. Garnish with smoked raspberries and a grilled lime wheel. Enjoy!

Smoked Pumpkin Spice Latte

Servings: 4

Cooking Time: 45 Minutes

Ingredients:

➢ 1 Small sugar pumpkin

➢ olive oil

➢ 1 Can sweetened condensed milk

➢ 1 Cup whole milk

➢ 2 Tablespoon Smoked Simple Syrup

➢ 1 Teaspoon pumpkin pie spice

➢ pinch of salt

➢ cinnamon

➢ whipped cream

➢ shaved nutmeg

➢ 8 Ounce smoked cold brew coffee

Directions:

1. Supply your smoker with wood pellets and follow the start-up procedure. Preheat the grill, with the lid closed, to 325° F.

2. Cut the sugar pumpkin in half, scoop out the seeds and discard. Place the pumpkin halves cut side up on a baking sheet and brush lightly with olive oil.

3. Place the sheet tray directly on the grill grate and cook 45 minutes or until the flesh is tender. Remove from heat and place on the counter to cool. Grill: 325 °F

4. When the pumpkin is cool enough to handle, scoop out the flesh and mash until smooth.

5. Place 3 Tbsp of the pumpkin puree in a separate bowl and reserve the remaining for another use.

6. Add the sweetened condensed milk, whole milk, Traeger Smoked Simple Syrup, pumpkin pie seasoning and salt to the pumpkin puree. Whisk to combine.

7. Pour the cold brew over ice, add desired amount of pumpkin spice creamer and top with whipped cream, cinnamon, and shaved nutmeg if desired. Enjoy!

Traeger Boulevardier Cocktail

Servings: 2

Cooking Time: 60 Minutes

Ingredients:

➢ 4 oranges

➢ 1/2 Cup honey

➢ 1500 mL rye whiskey

➢ 1 1/2 Ounce Campari

➢ 1 1/2 Ounce sweet vermouth

➢ 2 Tablespoon granulated sugar

➢ 3 Ounce grilled orange infused rye

Directions:

1. Supply your smoker with wood pellets and follow the start-up procedure. Preheat the grill, with the lid closed, to 350° F.

2. Slice 2 oranges in half and coat cut side with honey. Peel remaining orange and place peels on the grill. Cook 20 to 25 minutes. Grill: 350 °F

3. Remove from grill and let cool. Place orange halves cut side down directly on the grill grate and cook 20 to 30 minutes or until dark grill marks appear. Remove orange halves and allow to cool. Grill: 350 °F

4. Place orange halves into a bottle of rye whiskey and let steep for 10 to 12 hours. The longer they steep, the sweeter and more pronounced the orange flavor will be.

5. Add all ingredients into a mixing glass and stir until diluted. Strain into a fresh coupe glass and serve neat.

6. Garnish with grilled orange peel. Enjoy!

Grilled Blood Orange Mimosa

Servings: 4

Cooking Time: 15 Minutes

Ingredients:

➢ 3 blood orange, halved

➢ 2 Tablespoon granulated sugar

➢ 1 Bottle sparkling wine

➢ thyme sprigs, for garnish

Directions:

1. Supply your smoker with wood pellets and follow the start-up procedure. Preheat the grill, with the lid closed, to 375° F.

2. When the grill is hot, dip the cut side of the orange halves in sugar and place cut side down directly on the grill grate. Grill: 375 °F

3. Grill the oranges for 10-15 minutes or until grill marks develop. Grill: 375 °F

4. Remove from the grill and let cool at room temperature.

5. When cool enough to handle, juice the oranges and strain through a fine strainer removing any pulp.

6. Pour 5 oz of sparkling wine into each glass and top with 1 oz blood orange juice.

7. Garnish with a sprig of thyme. Enjoy!

BEEF LAMB AND GAME RECIPES

Beginner's Smoked Beef Brisket

Servings: 4

Cooking Time: 720 Minutes

Ingredients:

- 1 (6 lb) flat cut brisket, trimmed
- Beef Rub
- 2 Cup beef broth, beer or cola
- 1/4 Cup apple cider vinegar, apple cider or apple juice
- 2 Tablespoon Worcestershire sauce
- Texas Spicy BBQ Sauce

Directions:

1. Supply your smoker with wood pellets and follow the start-up procedure. Preheat the grill, with the lid closed, to 180° F.

2. Season on both sides with the Traeger Beef Rub.

3. Make the Mop Sauce: In a clean spray bottle combine the beef broth, beer or cola with apple cider vinegar and Worcestershire sauce.

4. Arrange the brisket fat-side down on the grill grate and smoke for 3 to 4 hours, spraying with the mop sauce every hour. Grill: 180 °F

5. Increase the grill temperature to 225°F and continue to cook, spraying occasionally with mop sauce, until an instant-read thermometer inserted in the thickest part of the meat reaches 204°F, this should take about 6 to 8 hours. Grill: 225 °F Probe: 204 °F

6. Foil the meat and let it rest for 30 minutes. Slice with a sharp knife across the grain into pencil-width slices. Serve with BBQ sauce. Enjoy!

Jalapeno Pepper Jack Cheese Bacon Burgers

Servings: 4

Cooking Time: 30 Minutes

Ingredients:

- ➤ 4 Slices, Raw Bacon
- ➤ 1/2 Cup Prepared Barbecue Sauce
- ➤ 1 Pound Ground Beef
- ➤ Hickory Bacon Seasoning, Plus More For Sprinkling
- ➤ 2 Thinly Sliced Jalapeno Peppers
- ➤ 1/2 Cup Olive Oil
- ➤ 4 Onion Burger Buns
- ➤ Onion, Crispy
- ➤ 4 Pepper Jack Cheese, Sliced

Directions:

1. Supply your smoker with wood pellets and follow the start-up procedure. Preheat the grill, with the lid closed, to 350° F. If using a gas or charcoal grill, set it up for medium high heat.

2. Make the burgers: in a large bowl, mix together the ground beef and Hickory Bacon seasoning until the seasoning is well incorporated. Use the Burger Press to make burger patties. Repeat until all the ground beef is gone.

3. In a small bowl, toss the sliced raw jalapenos with the olive oil and place them in the vegetable grill basket. Grill the jalapenos, stirring occasionally, until soft and charred in some spots. Remove from the grill and set aside.

4. Place the bacon on the vegetable grill basket and grill for 5-7 minutes, or until the bacon is crispy and brown. Remove from the grill and set aside.

5. Grill the burgers: place the burger patties on the grill and, if desired, sprinkle more Hickory Bacon seasoning on the patties. Grill the burgers for 5 minutes on one side, then flip and top with a slice of pepper jack cheese and grill for another 5-7 minutes, or until the internal temperature of the burgers is 135-140°F.

6. Remove the burgers from the grill and place on an onion bun. Top with the bacon, grilled jalapenos, crisped onions, and a spoonful of barbecue sauce.

Roasted Duck

Servings: 4

Cooking Time: 180 Minutes

Ingredients:

➢ 1 (5-6 lb) duck, defrosted

➢ Pork & Poultry Rub

➢ 1 Small onion, peeled and quartered

➢ 1 orange, quartered

➢ fresh herbs, such as parsley, sage or rosemary

Directions:

1. Remove the giblets and discard or save for another use. Trim any loose skin at the neck and remove excess fat from around the main cavity. Remove the wing tips if desired.

2. Rinse the duck under cold running water, inside and out, and dry with paper towels.

3. Prick the skin all over with the tip of a knife or the tines of a fork; do not pierce the meat. This helps to render the fat and crisp the skin.

4. Season the bird, inside and out, with Traeger Pork and Poultry Rub. Tuck the onion, orange, and fresh herbs into the cavity.

5. Tie the legs together with butcher's string.

6. Supply your smoker with wood pellets and follow the start-up procedure. Preheat the grill, with the lid closed, to 225° F.

7. Place the duck directly on the grill grate. Roast for 2-1/2 to 3 hours, or until the skin is brown and crisp. The internal temperature should register 160°F in the thigh (be sure to avoid the bone as this will give you an inaccurate reading). Grill: 225 °F Probe: 160 °F

8. If the duck is not browned to your liking, increase the grill temperature to 375°F and roast for several minutes at the higher temperature. Grill: 375 °F

9. Tent the duck loosely with foil and allow it to rest for 30 minutes.

10. Remove the butcher's twine and carve. Enjoy!

Smoked Meatball Egg Sandwiches

Servings: 4   Cooking Time: 25 Minutes

Ingredients:

- 3/4 Cup Breadcrumbs
- 2 Cloves Garlic, Minced
- 1 & 1/2 Lb. Ground Chuck
- 1 Jar Of Your Favorite Marinara Sauce
- 1 Large Eggs
- ¼ Cup Onion
- ¼ Cup Parsley, Minced Fresh
- ½ Tsp Pepper
- 1 Tbsp Chop House Steak Seasoning
- Provolone Cheese, Sliced
- ½ Tsp Salt
- Shredded Mozzarella Cheese
- 4 Sub Rolls Or Baguettes (6"), Sliced
- 2 Tbsp Worcestershire

Directions:

1. In a larger mixing bowl, combine the ground chuck, onions, garlic, Chop House Steak seasoning, salt, pepper, fresh parsley, Worcestershire, and egg. Add the breadcrumb mixture and parmesan cheese to the bowl and fold it into meat until well combined.

2. Supply your smoker with wood pellets and follow the start-up procedure. Preheat the grill, with the lid closed, to 400° F. If you're using a gas or charcoal grill, set it up for medium high heat and add your cast iron pan to the grill to warm up.

3. Roll the meat mixture into balls about 1 ½ inches wide, roughly the size of golf balls. Place meatballs into the cast iron skillet. Cook for 15 minutes or until meatballs are fully cooked and beginning to brown.

4. Pour full jar of marinara into the cast iron pan and gently stir to coat meatballs. Let simmer for 10-15 minutes.

5. Tear off four sheets of aluminum foil and place a sliced bun in the center of each. Divide the meatballs with sauce among the rolls. Top each roll with provolone cheese slices and mozzarella, and wrap entire sandwich tightly in foil. Return to the grill and cook an additional 10 minutes or until cheese is melty and bread has toasted. Serve immediately and enjoy!

Lamb Chopswith Lemon Vinaigrette

Servings: 4   Cooking Time: 16 Minutes

Ingredients:

- ➤ 8 lamb rib chops, about 2lb (1kg) total and each about ¾ inch (2cm) thick
- ➤ 3 tbsp extra virgin olive oil
- ➤ coarse salt
- ➤ freshly ground black pepper
- ➤ for the vinaigrette
- ➤ 4 lemons, halved
- ➤ 1 tbsp plus 1 cup extra virgin olive oil, plus more

- ➤ 4 large basil leaves, coarsely chopped
- ➤ 1 garlic clove, peeled and coarsely chopped
- ➤ 1 tsp Dijon mustard
- ➤ 1 tsp honey
- ➤ 1 tsp coarse salt
- ➤ ½ tsp freshly ground black pepper, plus more

Directions:

1. Supply your smoker with wood pellets and follow the start-up procedure. Preheat the grill, with the lid closed, to 450° F.

2. Coat the lamb chops on each side with the olive oil. Season with salt and pepper. (For the best crust, do this 45 minutes before grilling.)

3. Begin making the vinaigrette by brushing the lemon halves with 1 tablespoon of olive oil. Place the halves cut sides down on the grate and grill until they exhibit some charring, about 6 to 8 minutes. Transfer the lemons to a bowl and let cool.

4. Juice 4 lemon halves through a strainer positioned over a blender. (Reserve the remaining lemon halves for garnishing.) Add the basil leaves, garlic, mustard, honey, and salt and pepper to the blender. Add ¼ cup of olive oil and blend until the garlic is minced and everything's well combined. While the machine's running, slowly add the remaining ¾ cup of olive oil. Taste for seasoning, adding more salt. (If the dressing is too tart, add a little more honey or olive oil—the latter 1 tablespoon at a time.) Transfer the vinaigrette to a pitcher or a cruet.

5. Place the lamb chops on the still-hot grate at an angle to the bars. Grill until the chops have grill marks and the internal temperature reaches 125 to 135°F (52 to 57°C), about 3 to 4 minutes per side.

6. Transfer the chops to a platter and let rest for 3 minutes. Drizzle the lemon vinaigrette over the top. Place 1 reserved lemon half on each plate before serving.

Sweetheart Steak With Lobster Ceviche

Servings: 2

Cooking Time: 15 Minutes

Ingredients:

- 1 (20 Oz) Boneless Strip Steak Or Rib Steak, Butterflied Into Heart Shape
- 2 Teaspoon Jacobsen Salt Co. Pure Kosher Sea Salt
- 2 Teaspoon black pepper
- 2 Tablespoon Raw Dark Chocolate, finely chopped
- 1/2 Tablespoon olive oil
- 1 1/2 Pound Lobster Tail
- 1 Cup lemon juice
- 1/3 Cup lime juice
- 1/2 jalapeño, diced

Directions:

1. For the Sweetheart Steak, draw a large heart on a piece of cardboard, shape to size of meat selected. Cut out cardboard heart shape, then trim meat into heart shape.

2. Combine Jacobsen Salt, pepper, chocolate, and olive oil in a small bowl. Place on top of cut steak.

3. Cut raw lobster tail, remove meat, and chop. In a separate medium bowl, combine the lemon juice, lime juice, and jalapeno.

4. Toss in the lobster meat; ensure it is completely submerged in the liquid. Let lobster soak for 30 minutes. The citric acid actually cooks the lobster meat. If you prefer to have fully-cooked meat, grill lobster in shell for 3-5 minutes at 350 degrees F. Grill: 350 ℉

5. Remove from grill, then toss with lemon juice, lime juice, and jalapeno.

6. Supply your smoker with wood pellets and follow the start-up procedure. Preheat the grill, with the lid closed, to 450° F.

7. Place the steak directly on the grill grate and cook for 5 to 7 minutes per side, or until you've reached desired doneness. Remove from grill. Let rest for 5 minutes. Grill: 450 ℉

8. Serve lobster ceviche over steak. Enjoy!

Cucumber Beef Kefta

Servings: 4

Cooking Time: 10 Minutes

Ingredients:

➢ bamboo skewers, soaked in warm water

➢ 1 tbsp blackened saskatchewan rub seasoning

➢ 3 tbsp cilantro, chopped

➢ for topping, cucumbers

➢ 1 tsp cumin

➢ 2 lbs ground beef

➢ 1 tsp paprika

➢ 3 tbsp parsley, chopped

➢ pitas

➢ 1 red onion, grated

➢ for topping, tomatoes

➢ to taste, tzatziki sauce

Directions:

1. In a mixing bowl, combine ground beef, onion, Blackened Saskatchewan, cumin, paprika, cilantro, and parsley. Mix well, then cover and refrigerate for 1 hour to allow the flavors to blend.

2. Supply your smoker with wood pellets and follow the start-up procedure. Preheat the grill, with the lid closed, to 425° F. If using a gas or charcoal grill, set it up for medium-high heat.

3. Prepare kebabs: take small amounts of ground beef kefta and shape into popsicle-size cylinders. Skewer the meat, squeezing it to mold it to the skewer.

4. Grill kefta 3 to 5 minutes per side, then remove from the grill and serve warm with pitas, tzatziki sauce, and your favorite fresh veggies.

Standing Venison Rib Roast

Servings: 6

Cooking Time: 30 Minutes

Ingredients:

➢ 1 (2 To 2-1/2 Lb) 8-Bone Venison Roast

➢ 1 Tablespoon extra-virgin olive oil

➢ Prime Rib Rub

➢ Blackened Saskatchewan Rub

➢ Coffee Rub

Directions:

1. Supply your smoker with wood pellets and follow the start-up procedure. Preheat the grill, with the lid closed, to 375° F.

2. Rub the olive oil over the roast coating evenly. Then season with Traeger Prime Rib Rub liberally.

3. Place the roast directly on the grill grate bone side down.

4. Cook for 20-25 minutes or until the internal temperature reaches 125℉ when an instant read thermometer is inserted into the thickest part of the roast. Grill: 375 ℉ Probe: 125 ℉

5. Remove from the grill and let rest 5-10 minutes before carving. Enjoy!

Rosemary-smoked Lamb Chops

Servings: 4

Cooking Time: 125 Minutes

Ingredients:

➢ 4½ pounds bone-in lamb chops

➢ 2 tablespoons olive oil

➢ Salt

➢ Freshly ground black pepper

➢ 1 bunch fresh rosemary

Directions:

1. Supply your smoker with wood pellets and follow the start-up procedure. Preheat the grill, with the lid closed, to 180°F.

2. Rub the lamb chops all over with olive oil and season on both sides with salt and pepper.

3. Spread the rosemary directly on the grill grate, creating a surface area large enough for all the chops to rest on. Place the chops on the rosemary and smoke until they reach an internal temperature of 135°F.

4. Increase the grill's temperature to 450°F, remove the rosemary, and continue to cook the chops until their internal temperature reaches 145°F.

5. Remove the chops from the grill and let them rest for 5 minutes before serving.

Printed in the USA
CPSIA information can be obtained
at www.ICGtesting.com
LVHW082258180923
758602LV00007B/28